PILATES
FOR RUNNERS

HARRI ANGELL

BLOOMSBURY

LONDON • OXFORD • NEW YORK • NEW DELHI • SYDNEY

Bloomsbury Sport
An imprint of Bloomsbury Publishing Plc

50 Bedford Square
London
WC1B 3DP
UK

1385 Broadway
New York
NY 10018
USA

www.bloomsbury.com

BLOOMSBURY and the Diana logo are trademarks of Bloomsbury Publishing Plc

First published in 2017
Text © Harri Angell, 2016
Photos by Grant Pritchard

British Library Cataloguing-in-Publication Data
A catalogue record for this book is available from the British Library.

ISBN: Paperback: 9781472938008
ePub: 9781472938015
ePDF: 9781472938039

2 4 6 8 10 9 7 5 3 1

Designed by Susan McIntyre
Typeset in 11 on 14pt Myriad Pro Light Condensed
Printed and bound in China by Toppan Leefung Printing

Bloomsbury Publishing Plc makes every effort to ensure that the papers used in the manufacture
of our books are natural, recyclable products made from wood grown in well-managed forests.
Our manufacturing processes conform to the environmental regulations of the country of origin.

To find out more about our authors and books visit www.bloomsbury.com. Here you will
find extracts, author interviews, details of forthcoming events and the option to sign up for
our newsletters.

Contents

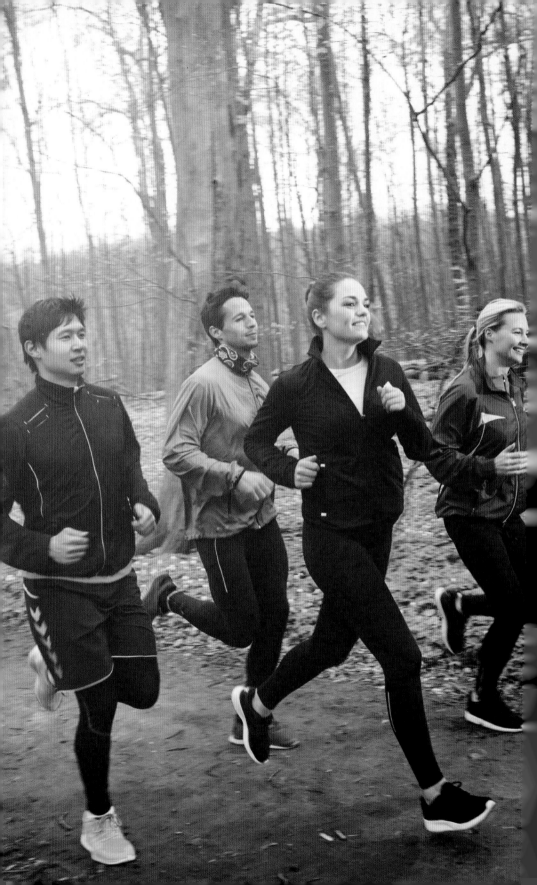

Introduction

This book is for anyone who runs.

Pilates can make a huge difference to your running form and help to keep you injury-free. Over time you will improve your strength, coordination, mobility, flexibility, breathing, balance and running posture – no more rounded shoulders or collapsed gait as you head for the finish line.

I have seen so many clients benefit in all sorts of positive ways from regular Pilates classes. And my own running form, stamina and times changed immeasurably once I started practising and then teaching it. Now, as I get older, I know that because of Pilates I can keep running comfortably for a long time to come. And by practising Pilates only a few times a week, I promise that you will also feel the difference, and maybe even notice that your body shape changes too.

In Chapter 2 I explain why Pilates is so beneficial for runners. This chapter will provide all the information needed to convince you to get started right away and to make this type of exercise part of your regular training. Whether you are male or female, a regular marathon runner, a Saturday morning parkrunner, a complete beginner or just contemplating taking up running, *Pilates for runners* is all you need to get the most out of this wonderful, life-enhancing sport and to stay injury-free.

You'll also find a whole range of exercises in the book to suit all levels of fitness ability, but before attempting them please do read Chapter 4 on postural alignment. Don't be tempted to skip chapters and jump straight to the exercises. While nearly all the exercises in this book stand alone, the information in Chapter 4 will give you the components needed to enable you to get the most out of your regular practice. And by applying some of the simple techniques outlined, you can begin to improve your posture before you even start exercising; you will notice a difference quite quickly.

Each of the exercises in this book starts with a brief explanation of the running benefits. I always need to know why I'm doing an exercise to fully understand how it works – so where possible there are explanatory notes. Not only will you learn how to perform the exercise, but also why you need to do it. This will give you added body awareness.

My intention is not to blind you with too much anatomy or biomechanical science, but to show you in the simplest, safest and most practical way how to execute the exercises in order to gain maximum benefit. If you feel discomfort, it goes without saying that you should stop

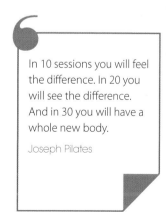

In 10 sessions you will feel the difference. In 20 you will see the difference. And in 30 you will have a whole new body.

Joseph Pilates

– you will recognize the difference between working muscles hard and something feeling not quite right. Listen to your body and work within your ability. Runners are prone to overdo their training, so take your time with the Pilates exercises, understand the reasoning behind them, follow the instructions and you can't go wrong.

In addition, throughout the book you will find motivating testimonials from all sorts of amazing runners – beginners and elite, young and not so young – who use Pilates as part of their training. There's also informative advice from professionals who advocate Pilates for runners, and a chapter on overtraining and injuries. Plus you'll find lots of inspirational quotes from the master himself, Joseph Pilates.

For too long there has been an air of mystery surrounding mat Pilates, or it has been thought of as an easy form of exercise only suitable for the elderly. My aim is to debunk these myths and to show you, the runner, that Pilates is a very precise and powerful fitness programme. It's actually quite magical! I look forward to encouraging more runners to give it a go, both men and women who until now haven't considered it as a relevant cross-training programme. I hope that through this book you too can discover how wonderful and accessible good, basic Pilates can be. It won't just change your running, it will change how you feel about yourself, and even your life. So pass it on!

Good luck – and happy, healthy running. Let me know how you get on.

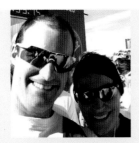

CASE STUDY

Andrew Strauss OBE and his wife Ruth McDonald ran the Virgin London Marathon in 2013 for The Lord's Taverners. Prior to that, Ruth had only ever run a 5k Race for Life, and Andrew had only run as a supplement to his cricket training. So once they reached the longer training runs their bodies began complaining, and they were advised to take up Pilates.

We started doing a Pilates session once a week and the difference it made to our bodies was evident and wonderful. We both became very aware of our strengths and weaknesses and were able to focus in on them during the session – and we were given homework! Ruth suffered from hip, knee and ankle discomfort and through Pilates her hip alignment and core strength improved and we both really felt that the Pilates kept us injury-free throughout our training. Actually the whole Pilates experience was good, not only physically but also mentally in the build up to the marathon. Pilates is a great way of challenging the body to be supple, strong and coordinated and we would recommend it to everyone. The Plank (page 69), the Side Bend (page 96), Teaser (page 149) and Hip Circles (page 132) targeted our needs perfectly! Race day was incredible and we would both say that we enjoyed the process of getting to the race day as much as the race itself, but we couldn't have done it without the Pilates.

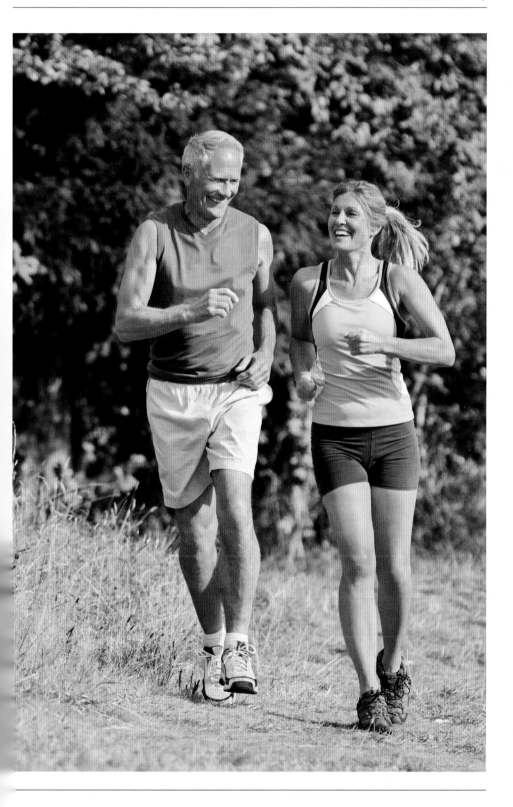

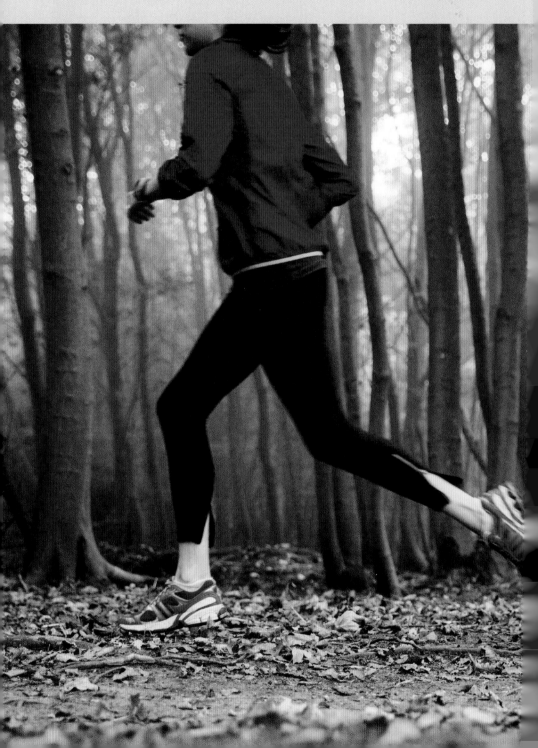

Chapter 1

Why Pilates is good for runners

Running is a repetitive activity. This means that every time you run you will be overusing some of your muscles, while others will be underused. Unfortunately, this overuse can cause muscular imbalances, which could turn into injury.

The repetitive nature of running causes your body to endure constant impact every time your feet hit the ground. The force of each stride travels up through your legs to the lower back and rib cage. If you have any weakness along the route of impact, this is where a problem can occur. So you need to make those vulnerable areas stronger and better able to deal with the stress of running. The Pilates exercises in this book will do this for you.

Think of your torso as the trunk and roots of a tree. They need a strong, solid foundation. If that trunk and its roots are weak, then the forces that the branches (your arms and legs) exert will uproot the tree, tip it over and break it. The same goes for your running body.

Pilates exercises are well known for improving core strength (the trunk and roots of the tree). They will make those vulnerable areas of your body better able to deal with the repetitive impact of running, increasing your running efficiency and therefore speed.

Along with core strength, Pilates improves your posture and body alignment. An upright body is a lighter body, which in turn will make you feel less tired because you are putting less strain on your musculoskeletal system.

> When all your muscles are properly developed, you will, as a matter of course, perform your work with minimum effort and maximum pleasure.
>
> Joseph Pilates

Think of your torso as the trunk and roots of a tree

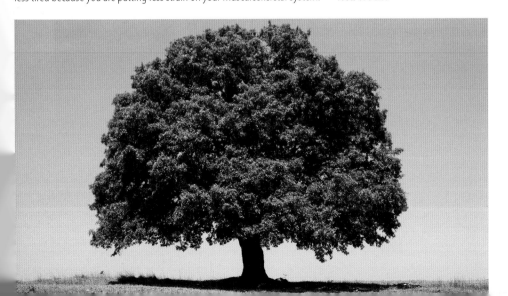

Core muscles

Abdominal muscles

In Pilates we talk a lot about the 'core' or the 'powerhouse', as the abdominal muscles are sometimes known. Your core is actually made up of a collection of different muscle groups: first of all the abdominal muscles, specifically the deepest, corset-like transversus abdominis muscle (TVA) that wraps around your middle between the lower ribs and the top of the pelvis. This works together with your pelvic floor muscles. And both these sets of muscles support the pelvis and spine by maintaining intra-abdominal pressure during any exertion, while allowing your limbs to move freely when you're running. If you suffer from back problems, it can often be because these muscles are weak (see lumbar spine, page 27).

At the side of your waist are your internal and external oblique muscles, and then on top of the deep TVA sits the more superficial rectus abdominis muscle, the potential 'six pack'. But it's the deep TVA that we are most interested in engaging and focusing on when performing Pilates exercises.

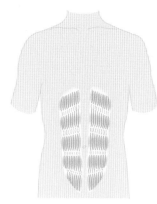

Rectus Abdominis

> I didn't realize how important core strength was until I got a strong core! It has paid off not only with my running but my everyday life: it affects how I sit, how I stand and run and I don't have a bad back – everything is just better with a strong core.
>
> Vassos Alexander, sports broadcaster, author and marathon runner

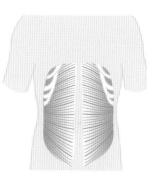

Transversus Abdominis

Glutes

Your glutes (buttock muscles) are also important core muscles – they need to be strong for you to run well and power up those hills. Maybe you've been told by your physiotherapist or osteopath that your glutes aren't firing? This is a good example of a muscle imbalance. If your glutes aren't doing their job, which is to stabilize your pelvis, the hamstrings (the muscles at the back of your thighs) take over the job and you start to suffer from tight hamstrings. See the Shoulder Bridge exercise on page 125 for some wonderful glute-strengthening exercises which will put you in touch with those muscles in a way that you never thought possible!

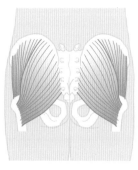

Glutes

Back muscles

A set of important back muscles, the multifidus and erector spinae are also part of the core. The multifidus works with the TVA and pelvic floor muscles to stabilize the pelvis and lower back. The erector spinae extends and laterally flexes the spine (side-to-side movement); it keeps the back straight and therefore influences your running posture.

All Pilates exercises work to strengthen and mobilize these really important running-efficient core muscles. These are the main stabilizers of the torso and lower limbs. They keep the trunk of the tree upright and strong and we need them to function well so that we can run comfortably to the best of our ability and remain injury-free. You'll find lots of back strengthening and lengthening exercises in this book.

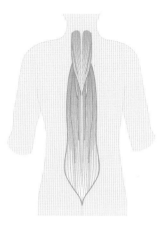

Erector spinae and multifidus

RESEARCH

Kimitake Sato and M. Mokha's research into core strength training and running at Barry University, Florida concluded that core strength training was indeed important in improving running speed and performance. The participants in their study completed a six-week core strength-training programme and experienced a significant improvement in their 5k times, as opposed to no increase in speed for the control group.

Balance and coordination

Balance

Runners need good balance. Think about how you run – one foot is off the ground with every stride you take. Have you ever tripped on uneven ground or turned your ankle? Maybe this is something you find happens regularly, especially if you are a trail runner and battling with tree roots or uneven paths.

In order to balance well, you have to *develop* balance, or proprioception (the ability to sense the position, location and orientation of your limbs in space).

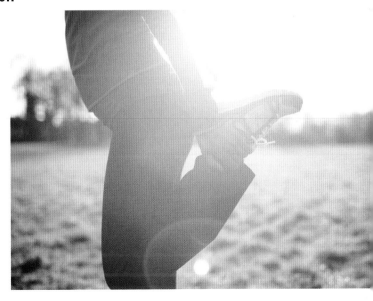

This skill doesn't just happen by magic, and unfortunately we begin to lose our ability to balance as we age. So it is essential that we keep practising it, and I suggest ways of doing this on page 55. If you're an off-road runner, potholes can appear from nowhere and be a real test of balance, especially if you are prone to tripping, as I used to be!

Coordination

As runners we need to coordinate our arm and leg movements and be conscious of our intentions, sometimes referred to as kinesthetic sensing (the ability to feel movements of the limbs and body). Remember the 'rub your tummy and pat your head' game? That's coordination. The better your coordination, the better your running agility, speed and power.

So you can see how important both good coordination and balance are for safe, injury-free, efficient running. Many of the mat Pilates exercises in this book will challenge and improve your balance and coordination skills, while they also work on your core strength.

RESEARCH

Proprioceptive/neuromuscular training (balance, coordination) was shown in a review of seven high-quality research studies by the Department of Sports Medicine, Goethe University, Frankfurt, to reduce incidence of lower limb injuries in sports that involve pivoting, running or jumping.

Breathing

Pilates will help to strengthen your diaphragm and improve posture – the more upright and open your chest when running, the easier it is to breathe when the going gets tough. When we become tired at the end of a run or race we tend to collapse from our centre, become round-shouldered shufflers and look down at the ground. This curved posture restricts the movement of the diaphragm and lungs.

Good lung capacity means that when you run you are able to transfer maximum oxygen into your body and muscles in order to optimize your ability. You need to be able to use your lungs fully and expand your rib cage comfortably, utilizing the diaphragm to power that breathing.

So practising the Pilates breathing, improving posture and strengthening the diaphragm will not only enhance your running style but also your general everyday well-being.

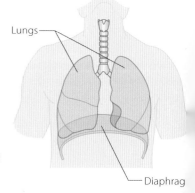

Lungs

Diaphrag

RESEARCH

According to Alison McConnell (PhD), we only use 50 to 60 per cent of our available lung capacity and rely heavily on our chest muscles when we breathe. Strengthening our diaphragms and breathing through the mouth when running can increase oxygen uptake.

Before any real benefit can be derived from physical exercises, one must first learn how to breathe properly. Our very life depends on it.

Joseph Pilates

Stretching

Post-exercise stretching is something some runners conveniently forget about. There is a lot of conflicting research out there about how important stretching actually is, but I believe it is vital. If the muscles remain shortened, not stretched, they become tight and weak, and injury can follow.

How many of you suffer from tight hamstrings or tight calf muscles after running? Do you just go and have a shower, or sit back down at your desk and don't move for hours? These bad habits shorten the hamstrings even more, and tight hamstrings will in turn shorten each of your running strides. Pilates improves flexibility by constantly lengthening the muscles during the exercises. In order that you can run well, you need your muscles to be long enough to withstand the full range of movement that this repetitive activity requires – think how many times these muscles have to contract.

RESEARCH

A 2011 study at the Faculty of Medical Sciences, Chiang Mai University by S. Phrompaet, A. Paungmali, U. Pirunsan and P. Sitilertpisan to assess and compare the effects of Pilates exercise on flexibility and lumbo-pelvic movement, showed that the Pilates training group improved flexibility significantly. This effect was also significantly greater than the control group for both four weeks and eight weeks of the training.

Posture

Pilates improves overall posture, and Chapter 4 is dedicated to postural alignment because it is such an important part of Pilates for runners. There are so many elements of posture to consider.

In brief, good posture – how you hold your body against gravity when running – is vital in order that you can run efficiently, with greater economy and with far less stress on the body. When your posture is good, there is literally less strain on the joints and bones because they are held in correct alignment. Muscles will remain lengthened and strong too. Your legs and arms will be free to work hard at propelling you comfortably forwards towards that race finish line and personal best, or in that gentle life-enhancing jog around the block.

> If your spine is inflexibly stiff at 30, you are old. If it is completely flexible at 60, you are young.
>
> Joseph Pilates

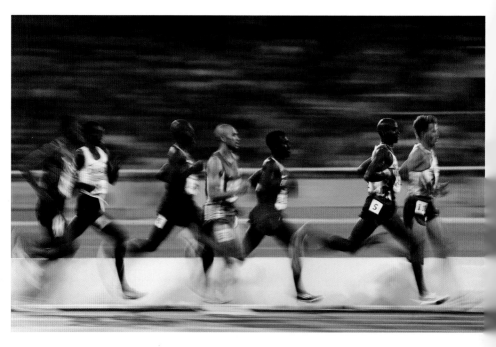

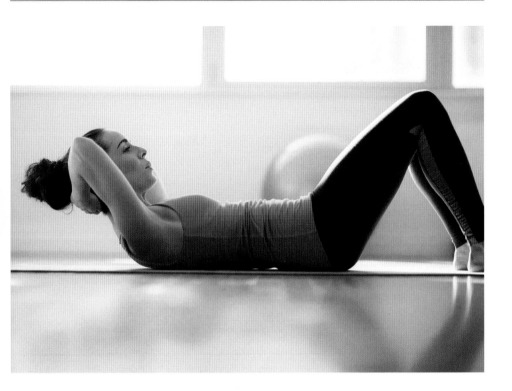

If you have ever overdone it on the abdominal work so that your muscles ache the next day, you will be aware that every single move you make requires a contribution from these important muscles. As well as these superficial 'main movers', the deeper postural and core muscles are also involved and required for everything from turning in bed to getting up off a chair. When it comes to running, these core muscles are vital in order to ensure that every aspect of your gait is executed in an appropriate way that will allow you to move efficiently without causing injury. With running, muscle imbalances can arise, for example the hip flexors can become tight and overpower the hip extensors (glutes). This means that the whole pelvic and hip complex is not working efficiently. Doing Pilates can help to address these imbalances, improving pelvic stability and keeping you injury-free. Because Pilates always works the right and left side of the body equally, and the front and back (or agonist and antagonist muscle groups), it can redress imbalances in muscle groups and improve postural alignment. I always recommend Pilates as the very best way to improve core strength.

Jane Kaushal, osteopath and runner

Chapter 2

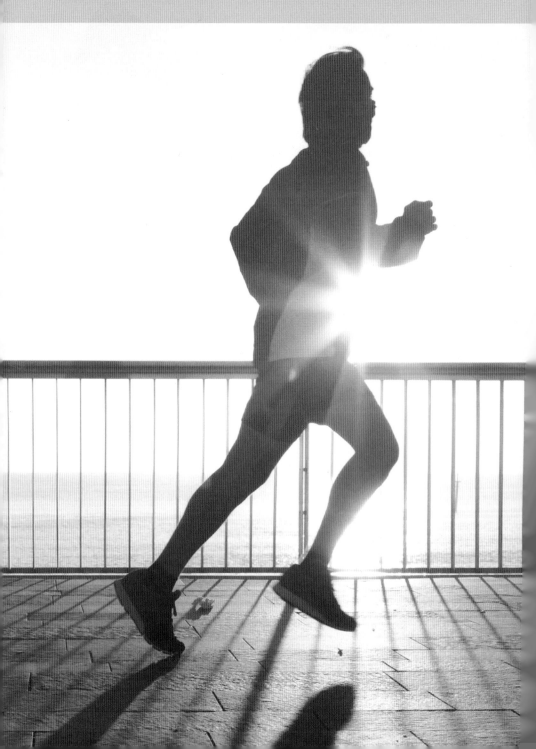

Joseph Pilates: a brief history

Joseph Hubertus Pilates was born in 1883 in Mönchengladbach, Germany, the second of nine children. As a child, raised in poverty, he suffered from rickets, asthma and rheumatic fever. Growing up he became frustrated by his frailty so started to explore ways to increase his physical fitness and improve his health. Leaving his sickly childhood behind, he became a gymnast, skier, boxer, diver and body builder, while also studying self-defence and meditation. As his body developed tone and shape, he even modelled for anatomy charts.

In 1912 Joseph Pilates moved to England and was employed to teach self-defence to members of the British police force and army; some biographies also claim that he was a circus performer at the same time.

When World War I broke out he was interned in Knockaloe Camp for German civilians on the Isle of Man. During his confinement he began to refine his exercise techniques, combining everything that he had learnt from yoga, gymnastics, self-defence, weight training and martial arts, and practised his exercise programme with his fellow inmates.

He called this method of body conditioning 'Contrology'. Joseph Pilates observed that if a body was misaligned or weak in a particular area, then muscles and joints would overcompensate in some way, often causing injuries. He continued to develop and refine his exercises, concentrating on physical remedies for postural misalignments.

> Contrology is complete coordination of body, mind and spirit designed to give you suppleness, natural grace and skill that will be unmistakably reflected in the way you walk, in the way you play, and in the way you work. You will develop muscular power with corresponding endurance, ability to perform arduous duties, to play strenuous games, to walk, run or travel for long distances without undue body fatigue or mental strain.
>
> Joseph Pilates, *Return to Life through Contrology*

After the war, Joseph Pilates returned to Germany. He taught self-defence to the Hamburg military police and the army and started working with Rudolph Laban (a dance artist and theorist), who introduced him to dance. In 1926, as a pacifist, Pilates became unhappy with the direction of German politics and decided to emigrate to America to join some of his relatives who were already living there.

On the ship travelling to America he met his future wife, Clara, who coincidentally shared his passion for fitness. Arriving in the USA, together they set up a fitness studio in a building shared with the New York City Ballet. They trained actors, dancers and athletes to develop core strength, and the Pilates method became well known for rehabilitating those with injuries. Martha Graham, considered the mother of modern dance, was an early devotee, along with George Balanchine, the choreographer who transformed the American ballet world.

By taking on apprentices and teaching them his programme of exercise, the Pilates method was passed on to others and continues to develop globally. Every health club in virtually every major city holds mat Pilates sessions today.

It is said that Joseph Pilates, always the showman, was often seen running the Manhattan streets in winter wearing just his signature white training pants. So it seems Pilates was in fact a runner too . . . although I wouldn't advocate the underpants look!

Joseph Pilates

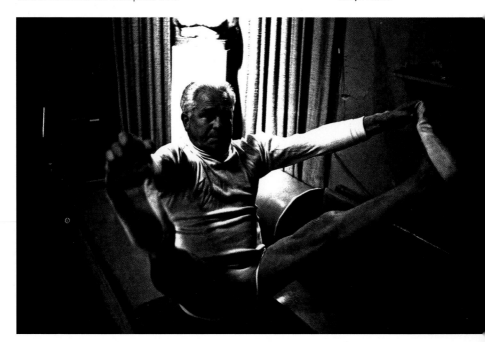

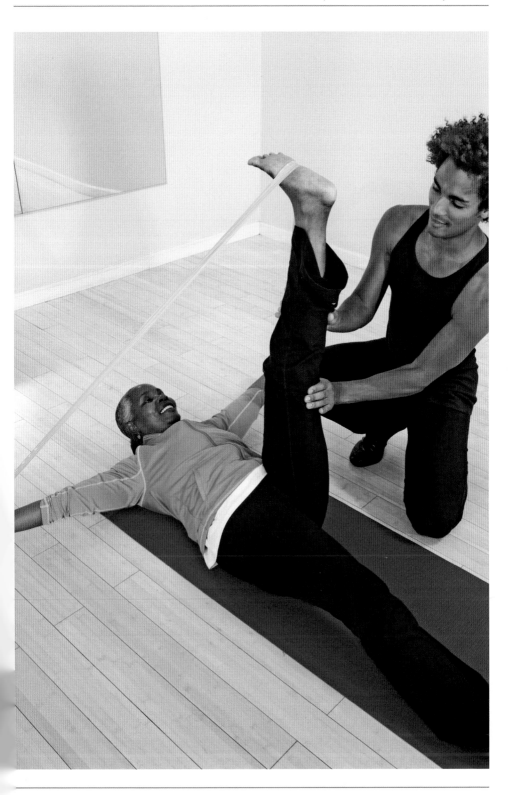

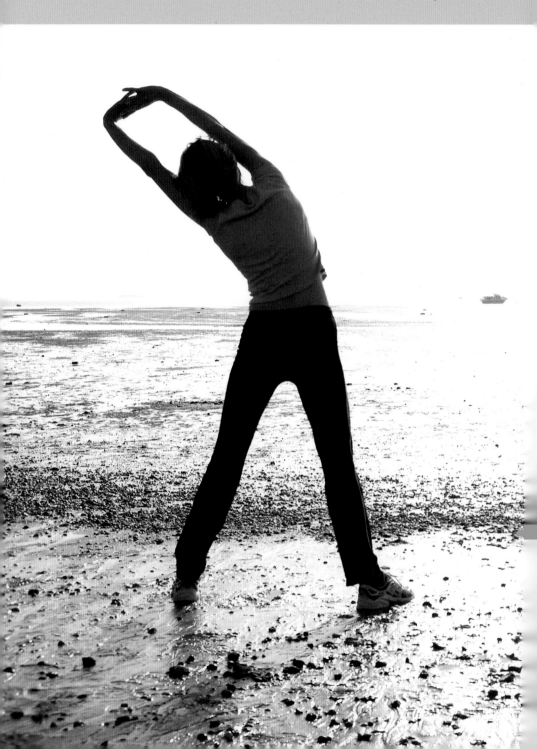

Chapter 3

The principles of Pilates

Joseph Pilates maintained that by following his exercise programme you could gain total control of your body. In addition he devised specific principles that he believed were necessary to accompany each of his exercises. Over the years different schools of Pilates have adapted these principles, or added a variety of others to the list, but all are still respectful of and relevant to the Pilates method.

For me, the following principles are worth acknowledging and applying when performing the exercises in this book. They can also, of course, be applied to your running.

Concentration

Being able to apply oneself wholly to the task in hand and block out any distractions isn't easy in our frenetic world. Once you are familiar with the exercises in this book you will find it easier to focus fully on each movement, allowing them to become flowing and connected. So try not to let your mind wander, ignore your 'to do' list, switch off your phone and instead begin to feel the connection between concentrating your mind and the movements of your body.

Eventually, with practice, the movement patterns will become second nature to you. Your concentration will improve and you'll begin to notice changes in the way you move and how you run.

I think mindfulness could also accompany this principle: performing the exercises, being at one with the moment, observing how it feels and paying attention to your body and its response.

Breathing

Quite simply, we need to breathe to live. But how well do we actually breathe? In Pilates the lateral thoracic breathing (page 37) helps the exercise to flow, aids concentration and allows the body to relax into the movement. If you're a breath-holder when you exercise you're not allowing

> Breathing is the first act of life, and the last.
>
> Joseph Pilates

your muscles to receive the oxygen that they need, which stresses the body and makes the movements more difficult, so it's worth trying to master the correct breathing technique at the same time as you learn the exercises. Pilates breathing is integral to the execution of the exercises and will strengthen your diaphragm, which in turn will improve your running strength and endurance.

Centring

'Core stability' is a modern term not coined by Joseph Pilates. Instead he referred to the core as the 'powerhouse' of the body. All Pilates exercises come from a strong centre: the core or powerhouse. By activating the deep transversus abdominis muscle (TVA) and pelvic floor muscles (page 32), we increase the overall strength and stability of the torso. Staying centred also refers to the mind: concentrating on the movement, being in the moment and focusing on what is happening in and to your body.

Alignment

Joseph Pilates called this 'precision': placing your muscles and joints in the correct, neutral position when performing the exercises. To read more about the neutral spine, see page 28. When the body is aligned from head to toe it's in its strongest position, where your muscles and joints can function optimally; this also applies to running. Pilates teaches you alignment through its emphasis on improving posture and you'll be checking your alignment before every exercise. Postural alignment is something you can start thinking about and apply immediately once you understand the process. When you next go out for a run you'll be thinking about it and feeling the difference in your technique.

Relaxation

Stay aware and recognize any tightness or tension that occurs in your body as you perform the exercises. Shoulders can rise up around the ears without you even realizing it, fists can be clenched and jaws locked. I see this all the time in my Pilates classes. Dealing with any tensions in the body means that eventually they will disappear, making it easier to execute the movements required. When you fully relax your body you will be slowing your heart rate down as well, which in turn will relieve stress. Reducing the tension in your body is a benefit that can transfer to running.

Flow

All the movements in Pilates are designed to flow smoothly and gently into each other as you lengthen and strengthen your muscles. When you first begin practising Pilates you might find that the movements can be a bit jerky or rigid as you get used to what you need to do, especially if you're still struggling with the breathing. Admittedly there's a lot to think about, but be patient and over time this will change. Once again, be aware of what your body is doing, stay connected to what's happening and you'll find the flow will come naturally. And once you've mastered the breathing it will make all the difference to how you produce fluid and fluent movements.

Endurance

By challenging your stability and regularly working your muscles when practising the Pilates exercises, as you increase the repetitions and try the progressions, you will be building strength and stamina. Including Pilates in your weekly routine will pay dividends. And of course this transfers to your running: the stronger you become, the more you'll build resistance to injury and be able to comfortably and safely sustain those running miles.

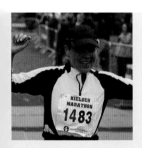

CASE STUDY

Alison Wolstenholme from Lancashire has been running for 10 years. She runs for pleasure, to keep fit and healthy and has run 11 marathons. Her favourite races are the Isle of Skye Half Marathon and Kielder Water Marathon. She attends a mat Pilates class once a week.

Since taking up Pilates I have greater flexibility and I run stronger. The breathing exercises have helped me develop a better breathing pattern and rhythm, and the Pilates exercises have helped my uphill running and strengthened my core, which means less pressure on my lower back. They've also strengthened my quads and hip abductors which helps support and protect my knees and hips when running. Pilates makes me think more about how I stand, walk and sit – I've really noticed that I now have a stronger and straighter spine. I always stretch after a run, but Pilates does a really good all-over body stretch and covers areas that I don't do immediately after a run. I know people who hardly ever stretch and they seem more susceptible to injury. I specifically signed up for classes on a Monday so that when I get into 'long-run' territory on a Sunday I have a Pilates session the next day. By doing the class the day after it gives me a full body stretch after all the high impact of big miles. Pilates helps to clear the mind of the everyday rubbish in my head too. I feel refreshed and ready to go again.

Chapter 4

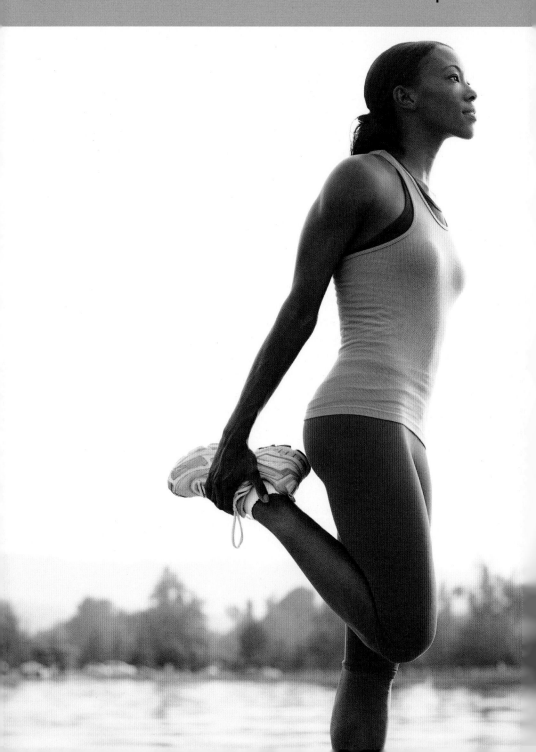

Postural alignment

If you've ever been a spectator at a race you will probably have seen all sorts of interesting running postures cross the finish line: rounded shoulders, chins poking forwards, knocking knees, twisting torsos, flailing arms – you name it, they're usually all there. And how often do you finish a race or run with a sore lower back, screaming hamstrings or tense shoulders? Hopefully not that often, but if you do, then by practising Pilates you will strengthen the muscles that cause these problems, and quite quickly you'll feel an improvement in your running form.

With a good, healthy, upright posture you will easily become a better runner. You'll finish with more energy in the tank because you can run taller, breathe more deeply, be lighter on your feet. Take a look at some of the elite runners' postures, how graceful and upright they are. Poor posture really does place stress on your body and sap energy. If left uncorrected this can lead to injury.

By observing your own or someone else's posture and movement you can often tell a lot about their personality or lifestyle. If you work in front of a computer, day in, day out, then maybe you have a tendency to rounded shoulders and you'll find you probably have tight hip flexors as well. If you cross your legs; if your computer isn't at eye level; if you always carry your baby only on your right hip; if you feel unhappy or in pain; if you wear high heels – everything can affect your posture. In addition, anxieties can turn into tension and unresolved emotions manifest in stress-related injuries, so it's not surprising that we end up with a body that compensates and then starts complaining.

It can also affect our well-being and reflect our emotions: standing upright, lengthening through the spine with an open chest and relaxed shoulders immediately feels better than being slouched and scrunched up in a 'miserable', collapsed stance.

As we age our posture changes too, so it's important to start looking after it and being body aware as early as possible. With good posture all your vital organs will be held in the right place, everything will function well and you will move so much more easily as you run to that finish line. And Pilates will start sorting it out right away.

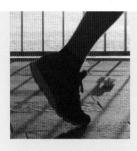

PROFESSIONAL ADVICE

Simon Poole, podiatrist, sees many runners in his clinic.

Our jobs, hobbies, daily commute can all place our bodies in positions that cause stress. Some structures will be overworked while others become underworked and weaker. Many people sitting at a desk slouch or sit with rounded shoulders, which over time can cause poor posture when running. Making sure that you have a well set up workspace is a great way to reduce this stress, but in a lot of cases they can't be totally eliminated and attending a Pilates class to improve posture can counter the effects of poor posture. As an interesting aside, a large number of female patients will often have a shoulder which is higher on one side than the other. In the clinic I will assess with gait analysis to see if it is as a result of a difference in the length of someone's legs or it may be a result of a curvature in the spine. But often after assessing, these are not present and it's as a result of the patient always carrying a bag on that shoulder. A simple day-to-day habit, but one which can greatly affect posture and function. Pilates can be a great way of reducing the effects.

The spine

When we walk or run our bodies are supported by the spine. It keeps us upright and carries the weight of our head, torso and arms. The impact the spinal column has to endure as we pound the ground is huge. Good running posture, learning to keep the spine in its strongest, safest position with the least stress placed on discs and ligaments will make all the difference, not only to your running but also to injury prevention. In addition, standing, walking or running with a lengthened spine makes you feel lighter and can have a positive effect on the psyche. It really can improve how you feel: slouching in a negative 'I can't do this run' mode, or lengthening and breathing openly in a positive 'I can do this!' mode? It's a no-brainer!

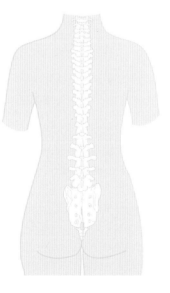
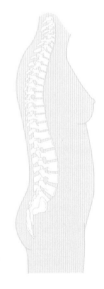

A normal spine

Lumbar spine

This is your lower back and where most back problems occur, which is not surprising as it acts as a shock absorber. If your abdominal muscles are weak then it's possible that they are not doing their job of keeping this part of your back protected. The TVA, which acts like a corset, wrapping itself around our middle (page 10), if not 'laced up properly' can allow the abdominal muscles to fall forwards. So strengthening the abdominal muscles and 'lacing up the corset' is vital for a healthy lower back.

Lordosis is the name given to an excessive curvature or arch of the lower back. Consequently, this type of posture can sometimes mean that there is an imbalance between your hip flexors – for example, one might be tighter and shorter than the other. Your lower back, hamstrings and inner thigh muscles might also feel tight, while your glutes and rectus abdominis are lengthened and therefore potentially weak. 'Flat back' posture is where there is little mobility in the lower back and the lumbar spine is flat. With this type of posture you'll find that the hamstrings and rectus abdominis are tight and the hips flexors tend to be long and weak.

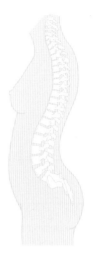

Lordosis

Thoracic spine

This is the middle of your back that can morph into a round-shouldered hunch. Many of the exercises in this book talk about strengthening or mobilizing the thoracic spine. However, in reality it's not a very mobile part of the back. It's important to us as runners because this part of our back supports the chest and rib cage, which moves as we breathe in and out. It also provides added support to our heads, which generally weigh around 4.5kg – so if alignment isn't quite right, then this part of our back and the areas it supports will suffer and so will our running.

Kyphosis is a condition in which the upper back curves excessively and the shoulders are rounded. This type of posture can mean that your pectorals (chest muscles) and rectus abdominis (six pack) are very tight, but that your lower trapezius muscles (upper back) and deltoids (shoulder) are long. This type of posture can be common in runners as this is often the position adopted over long distances when fatigued. Also, if you work in an office and sit at a desk all day, or if you are very tall, you might be familiar with this hunched, round-shouldered posture.

'Sway back' posture can be recognized by the increased curvature of the thoracic spine (kyphosis) as well as the lower lumbar spine which looks flat. The cervical spine (upper back/neck) is also slightly flexed and the head and chin tends to jut out. Generally this type of posture means that the hip flexors can be weak and lengthened, the upper rectus abdominis

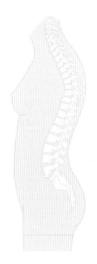

Kyphosis

and also the oblique (waist) muscles can be weak. In addition, sometimes the hamstrings can be short and the knee joints hyper-extended.

Over time, Pilates exercises will encourage the awareness to help you improve and go some way to correcting these postural imbalances. In turn this will have a positive effect on your running form along with any post-run aches and pains you might be suffering from as a result. But the first thing you need to do is familiarize yourself with your own posture, so that you can work on improving it. As you progress you will notice the difference that Pilates has made.

Alignment is everything. Throughout all the exercises in this book we are working on postural alignment, whether lying on your front, back, side or standing.

The following information is essential to be able to understand the Pilates exercises. You may need to keep referring back. Please read through the whole section to begin with, take a look at the pictures and then have a practice; not only will your posture start to improve right away, but the exercises will be easier to execute. It might help to have someone read out the following information when you perform the movements for the first time.

Neutral spine

All Pilates exercises start from neutral spine. Neutral spine is a good, strong, healthy position where the spine is lengthened in its natural curves.

Neutral spine when lying down on your back
This is the position in which your spine and pelvis are aligned and arranged in their strongest position with the least amount of stress placed on the discs and ligaments.

- To familiarize yourself with this position, lie on your back, bend your knees and place your feet parallel and in line with your hips.
- Take your arms down by your sides.
- Now tilt your pelvis backwards and forwards a few times, producing a pronounced arch under your lower back, then flattening your spine down on to the floor.
- These are exaggerated moves; neutral spine is the middle position between the two.
- This position should be relaxed, not forced and feel natural.

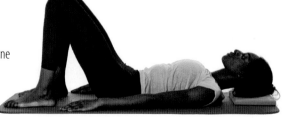

Neutral spine when standing up

- Stand tall, spine lengthened, with your feet in line with your hips.
- Place your hands on your hips.
- Rock your pelvis backwards and forwards – feel the movement under your hands.

- Imagine your pelvis is a bowl of water.
- When you tilt your pelvis forwards, the water from the bowl spills out the front.
- When you tilt your pelvis backwards the water from the bowl spills out the back.
- Bring the pelvis/bowl to the centre position where the water stays level and doesn't spill. That's neutral spine.

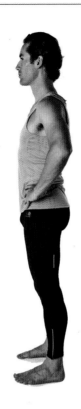
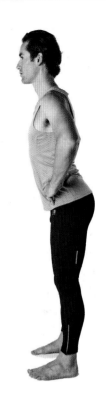

Throughout the exercises in this book I suggest 'pelvic tilts' as a way of finding your neutral spine – this is the action of moving your pelvis backwards and forwards, as described. It's also a great, simple exercise for a tight back after a run or if you've been sitting for too long.

Standing tall

During the warm-up sequence to the Pilates exercises it's important to take some time to learn how to stand tall and remain centred. This will transfer to your running technique and also your everyday life. If you can stand in front of a long mirror when you do the warm up it will give you a better idea of your posture, what needs to happen to improve it and what good posture looks like.

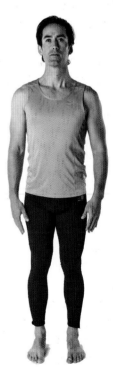

- Take a good look at how you stand.
- Does your head tilt a little to one side?
- Are your shoulders level or is one higher than the other?
- Are your hips level?
- Is your weight evenly distributed between your feet or are you leaning slightly?

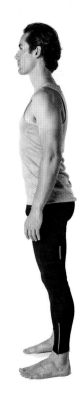

- Stand sideways and take a look at your lower back. Does it arch? (See lumbar spine, page 27.)
- Look at the middle of your back. Is it rounded? (See thoracic spine, page 27.)
- Does your chin jut out?
- Do you have rounded shoulders?
- Is your chest elevated in a military stance?
- Experts sometimes use what's called a 'plumb line' when taking a look at posture from the side. This is the line of gravity that runs vertically from your ear lobe down to the outside of your ankle bone.
- Once you have become familiar with your own postural alignment, turn back to face the mirror.
- Place your feet directly below your hips and make sure that they are facing forwards – not turned out at ten-to-two or toe to toe. Your weight should be evenly distributed.
- Notice whether your knees are above your ankles – sometimes knees come together a little; if yours do, be aware of this.
- Hips should be placed above the knees.
- Relax your arms by your sides.
- Lengthen through your spine, imagining you have a big bunch of helium balloons attached to the top of your head lifting you upwards – notice how you immediately grow taller and feel lighter.
- Keep this lengthening in your spine. Don't forget to lengthen your neck too.
- Your chin should be parallel to the floor and your gaze focused straight ahead.
- Relax your shoulders.
- Relax your jaw.
- Notice the changes and how different you feel.

Standing also is very important and should be practised at all times until it is mastered … never slouch, as doing so compresses the lungs, overcrowds other vital organs, rounds the back and throws off the balance.

Joseph Pilates

Running posture

- When you're running, lengthen your spine upwards, as described on page 30; this naturally brings your spine and pelvis into neutral or nearly neutral alignment.
- If you're tired, then your torso might tend to collapse at its centre and your spine begin to sag so that you lose that neutral position. Visualize those helium balloons attached to the top of your head, lifting you upwards as you run. Feel light on your feet as you propel yourself forwards.
- Another useful visualization is imagining you have a bungee attached to the middle of your chest, pulling you forwards towards your destination. Keep your focus on something in the distance just a little higher than your eyeline, feeling upright and light as you run comfortably with spine lengthened and spirit lifted!

Engaging the abdominal muscles and pelvic floor muscles

When you perform the Pilates exercises in this book you will need to engage your deep abdominal muscles (TVA) and/or your pelvic floor muscles before you move. When you first start practising Pilates it can be hard to do both at the same time, so although in the exercises I mention both, choose one – take your time to experiment and get to know how each contraction feels and what difference they make to the execution of the exercises and your running.

The following visualization and exercise will demonstrate how to do this, and once again it's something that you can start practising straight away: in the supermarket queue, at the bus stop, walking the dog and, of course, running those wonderful miles.

Abdominal muscles

- Imagine you have a big belt wrapped around your waist. The belt has 10 notches.
- Visualize pulling the belt to the tenth notch so that your abdominal muscles are pulled right in as far as they will go – not very comfortable!
- Relax.
- Now pull the belt to the fifth notch.
- A little more comfortable for your abdominal muscles.
- Relax.
- Now pull the belt to the third notch.
- And that's where you want to be pulling your abdominal muscles in to each time you perform an exercise. Try to reach the third notch on your imaginary belt.

When you are pulling your abdominal muscles in you are supporting and stabilizing your spine, immediately making your torso stronger. Try doing this when you run too, keeping those abdominal muscles activated for as long as possible. You will immediately run stronger and feel a difference.

Pelvic floor muscles

Alongside the TVA, the pelvic floor muscles work to help stabilize and support the spine and pelvis by maintaining intra-abdominal pressure during any exertion. Running obviously increases this intra-abdominal pressure, so a weak pelvic floor can lead to all sorts of problems for both men and women.

Pilates exercises are an excellent way to strengthen the pelvic floor muscles, and if yours are weak and you have problems as a result, these exercises will begin to sort you out.

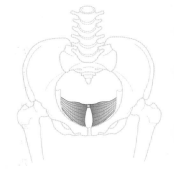

Your pelvic floor muscles

- To contract your pelvic floor muscles, the simplest way to describe it is to imagine stopping the flow of urine when you go for a wee! This applies to both men and women.
- And notice as you pull your pelvic floor muscles up how your abdominal muscles activate at the same time – proof, if you need it, that these two sets of muscles work together to support the spine and stabilize the pelvis.

The pelvic floor is a sheet of muscle and connective tissue that spans the area underneath the pelvis, providing support to the pelvic organs including the bladder, intestines and, in women, the womb. There is good evidence that pelvic floor exercises are beneficial in the management of urinary incontinence in women and are used as a first line of treatment before other options such as surgery are considered. Pelvic floor strengthening is particularly useful with 'stress incontinence', which is where leakage of urine occurs with coughing, sneezing, jumping, or any activity that leads to a rise in pressure in the abdomen. Women also report that they leak urine when running and sadly this can lead to them avoiding this and other physical activities. Up to 70 per cent improvement can be seen in symptoms when exercises are done correctly and consistently. Having an awareness of your pelvic floor through practising Pilates and the benefits of strengthening and pulling up that muscle 'sling' will lift the pelvic organs and keep them where they are meant to be and work best. So as well as strengthening all the other muscles that you need in order to run well and safely, Pilates can also help you to remain continent while doing so!

Dr Helen Kennedy, GP, with a special interest in women's health

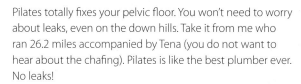

Pilates totally fixes your pelvic floor. You won't need to worry about leaks, even on the down hills. Take it from me who ran 26.2 miles accompanied by Tena (you do not want to hear about the chafing). Pilates is like the best plumber ever. No leaks!

Fiona O'Donovan, parkrunner, 10k, half marathon and marathon runner

Shoulder stabilization

Maintaining shoulder stabilization during Pilates exercises is another important part of postural alignment. An awareness of what your shoulders are doing will help you to perform the exercises without them becoming tense and inadvertently ending up around your ears. If you suffer from tight shoulders, this will help relieve the tension.

- Lift both your shoulders right up to your ears.
- Take them backwards and down – imagine your shoulder blades sliding down into the back pockets of your trousers.
- Relax your shoulders for a moment and then repeat a few more times, lifting up to your ears and then sliding your shoulder blades down.
- This is a great way to open out the chest and help the shoulders relax – something you can perform if you've been sitting hunched over your desk for a long time or driving for hours. Or try it before you start a race if you're suffering from 'race nerves' and feeling tense.

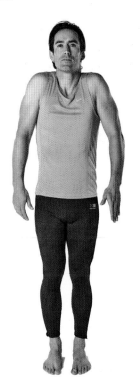
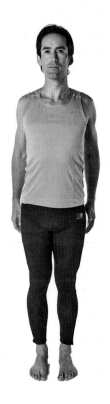

(For more on suggested pre-race relaxing rituals, see page 196.)

Imprinting the spine

Imprinting the spine ensures spinal stability when both your feet are lifted off the ground. If finding neutral spine is a challenge and your abdominal muscles don't feel strong enough to support your spine, then it can be advisable to imprint the spine before you move into the tabletop position (see The Hundred exercise, page 116).

- Lie on your back, knees bent with your feet in line with your hips.

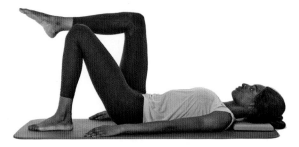

- Engage your abdominal muscles and sink your back very gently down into the floor 'imprinting' it on the mat. Raise one leg into the tabletop position.

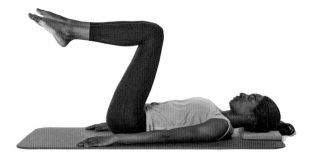

- Raise the other leg up into the tabletop position to join it.

- This 'imprinting' position is all about ensuring that your back is in a safe position when your legs are raised if you're unable to sustain neutral spine.
- If you have a serious back problem please consult your medical practitioner to check that this position is safe for your particular condition.

> When I started to get back problems I feared that I would have to stop running. Then I discovered Pilates. Running without core strength puts strain on the spine and this was the cause of my back problems. After a few months of Pilates I could feel the difference and was soon able to return to running. Pilates has so many added benefits – I noticed an improvement in balance, breathing and concentration. Now I am thrilled to be training for a half marathon.
>
> Deanne Ashman, recreational runner

Chapter 5

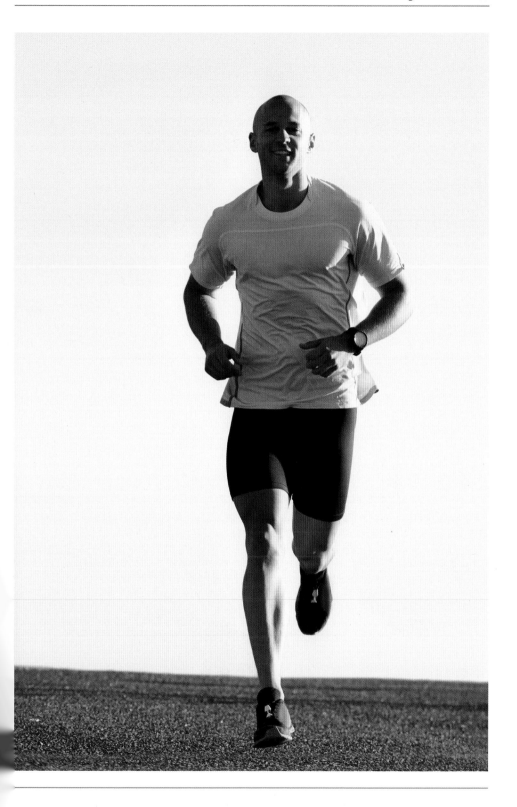

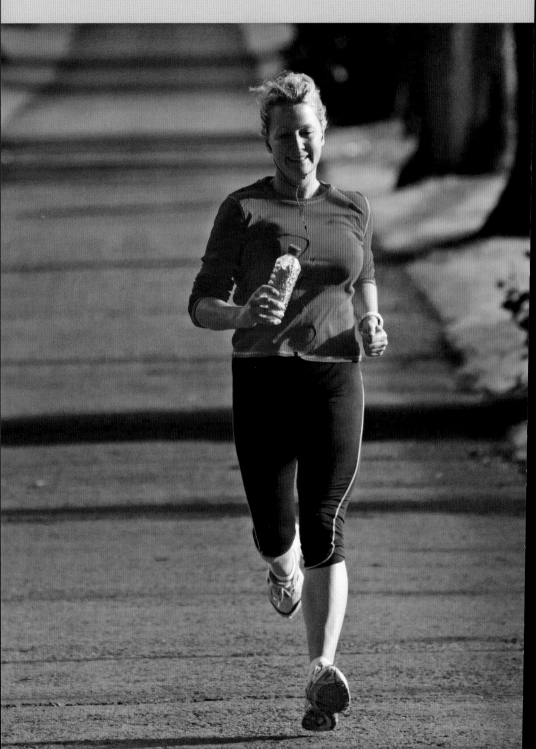

Breathing

Pilates breathing

Pilates breathing is known as 'lateral thoracic breathing'.

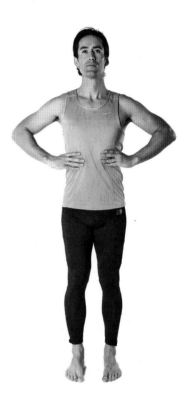

- Stand tall and lengthen through your spine.
- Breathe in deeply, through your nose, into your rib cage, and then slowly breathe out through your mouth.
- The reason we do this lateral thoracic breathing into the rib cage and not into the abdominal cavity is so that you can activate your abdominal muscles at the same time as breathing – if you were belly breathing it would be quite challenging to pull the abdominal muscles in.
- Practise this breathing a few times.
- Place your hands either side of your torso on your rib cage.
- Breathe in through the nose and feel how the rib cage expands underneath your hands.
- Breathe out slowly through your mouth and allow your rib cage to relax.
- Try not to let your shoulders rise up as you breathe.
- This type of breathing is just for the Pilates exercises as it helps the exercises to flow, strengthens your diaphragm and encourages you to relax the body.
- For some people this is the hardest part of practising Pilates, so take your time if you find the lateral thoracic breathing challenging. Try it out every now and again, and slowly you will find yourself getting into the rhythm of it.
- Whatever happens, just remember to breathe when you perform the exercises – don't hold your breath!

Running breathing

I'm often asked by new runners how to breathe correctly when running. Obviously we want to get as much oxygen to the muscles as possible, and the quickest way to do that is by breathing through the mouth, which happens automatically. However, there are lots of differing opinions about how to breathe when you run. Whichever way you do choose to breathe, make sure you are breathing into your diaphragm, letting it expand and contract as you do so, rather than breathing into your chest, because this is a shallow way to breathe and therefore inefficient.

When you first start to run, the temptation is to go too fast, before your heart and lungs have had time to adapt. This means that you will be out of breath. The only way to change this is to slow down and wait until your body is ready to speed up, then it will all fall into place naturally.

Lateral thoracic breathing, the breathing we adopt in Pilates, will strengthen your diaphragm, which does 80 per cent of the breathing work. We can't make our lungs any bigger but we can improve our posture to help those lungs and our diaphragms function more efficiently, which in turn will improve our running endurance.

Chapter 6

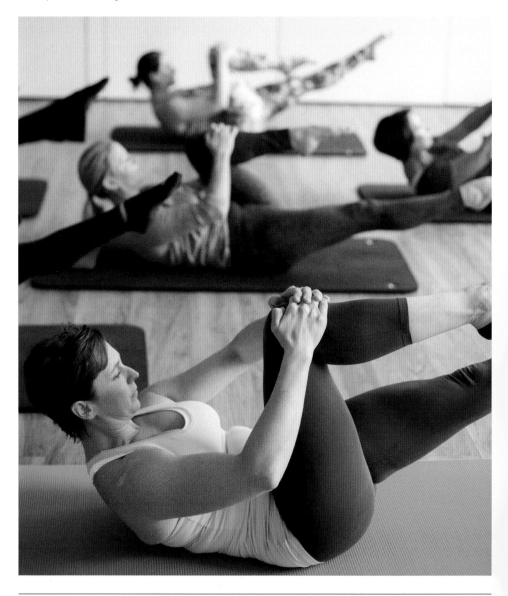

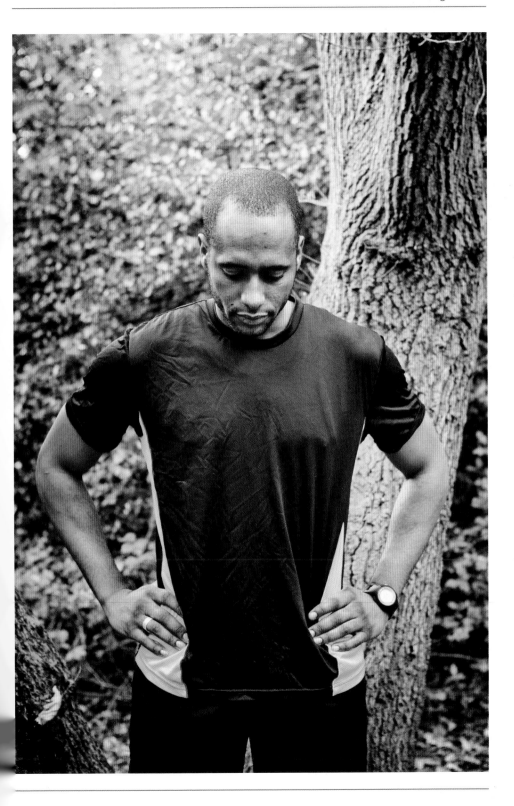

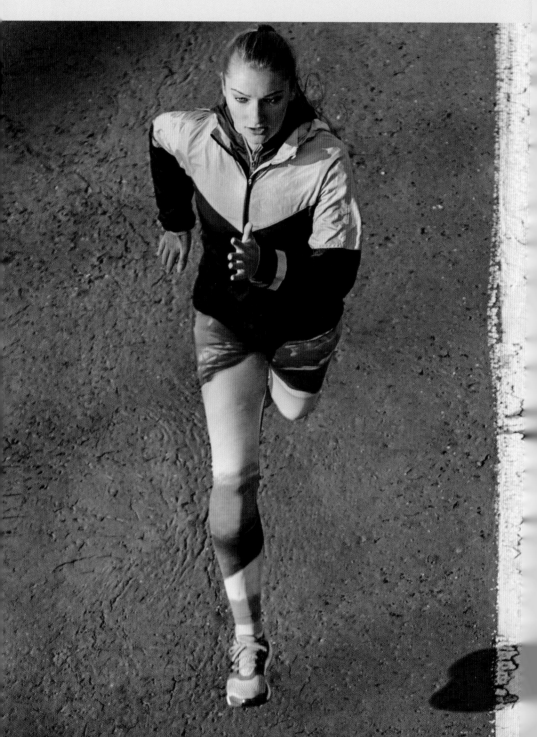

Equipment

Pilates, in general, just requires a mat. Having said that, I have chosen to include some extra equipment in some of the exercises to make them more challenging. It's up to you whether you choose to include these in your weekly programme or not. So before you start practising the exercises in this book it's a good idea to get yourself prepared. Wear comfortable clothes in which you can move around freely – running kit is perfect – and make sure you have enough space around you. Ideally, all exercises should be performed in bare feet or socks.

- A Pilates or yoga mat makes for a more comfortable experience. You will need some cushioning, especially when lying on your front, side or rolling. There are different types of mats on the market, but I would suggest one of the thicker sort so that your spine and joints are better protected. If you practise your Pilates on a hard rather than carpeted floor, you will need to make sure you have a mat that won't slip and that your hands and feet can grip on to as well.

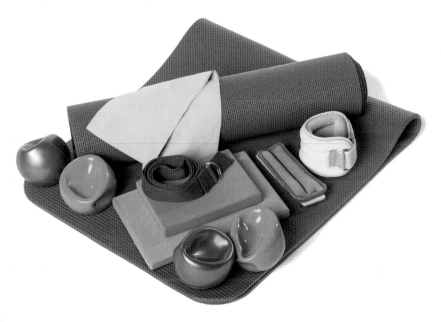

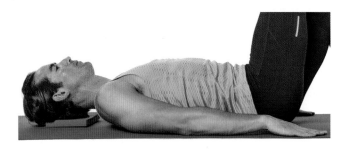

- A small, firm foam block (20 × 15 × 2cm) is useful, or you can use a rolled-up towel or small cushion to put under your head, so that your neck and spine stay aligned. Obviously everyone's posture is different, so you will need to experiment with this. If you find that your head tilts back, sending your chin into the air when lying down flat with nothing supporting your head, then place the block underneath to bring your neck into alignment. If, however, the opposite happens and your chin comes forwards on to your chest when you place your head on the block, then don't use one. Think about placement – are your neck and spine aligned? – and then adjust accordingly.

- Dyna-Bands™ or yoga straps for stretching and hip circles are cheap and versatile pieces of kit.

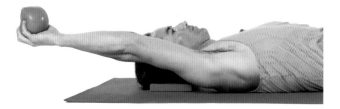

- Small hand weights are an excellent addition but are, of course, optional. In some of the exercise progressions I make suggestions about when you might like to use light hand weights. In my classes we use soft ball-shaped weights which are safer than the hard ones for these type of exercises. Or you can make your own by filling small plastic water bottles with sand or water.

- Ankle weights – again, these are optional and in some of the Side Series progressions I have suggested (pages 88–99) you might want to use them to increase the challenge.

Note: *it's important that you can execute the exercises in a flowing, smooth fashion, keeping correct alignment throughout, before adding in any weights.*

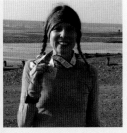

CASE STUDY

Sarah Sawyer is a runner and Pilates teacher from Brighton who runs everything from 5ks to 100-mile ultra marathons and everything in between. She's run all over the world and some of her favourite places to run are Jordan, Ecuador and the French Alps. Closer to home she loves running on the South Downs.

I started running about six and a half years ago and I've run about 25 marathons/ultras and then lots of shorter races on road (5ks, 10ks and half marathons). I've done a couple of multi-stage races in the desert in Jordan and through the Andes in Ecuador, where I've run 155 miles over six stages carrying everything I need on my back – as you can imagine, a strong core has been my saviour when you're carrying 8kg of food, sleeping equipment and kit on your back!

I started practising Pilates at the same time as I started running. So many articles tell runners to complement their running with Pilates … and most people ignore it! However, I followed the advice and have been practising regularly ever since, and I credit Pilates massively with the fact that in all the time I've been running, I've never had an injury. I decided to do my Pilates training about two years ago, initially with the view to just improve my own practice and gain a deeper understanding of Pilates and how the body works. I qualified last year and started doing some teaching cover immediately. The feedback I received was really positive so I decided to set up my own 'Pilates for Runners' classes and they've been a real success and it's so rewarding seeing students similarly credit Pilates for keeping them injury-free as they're training for their races.

I see people who run much less than me being plagued with running injuries and I think it's because they don't supplement their running with anything else, so they'll have a weak core, weak glutes, tight hips etc! Personally, Pilates has made me so much stronger – I've never gone to a gym but regular mat classes have given me so much core strength which I believe is vital in running, especially when I'm running marathon distance and above, and off-road. Also without Pilates, I certainly wouldn't have had the strength to carry an 8kg rucksack on my back in my multi-day races. I also notice my running form is much better, especially towards the end of races when your body starts to tire.

Chapter 7

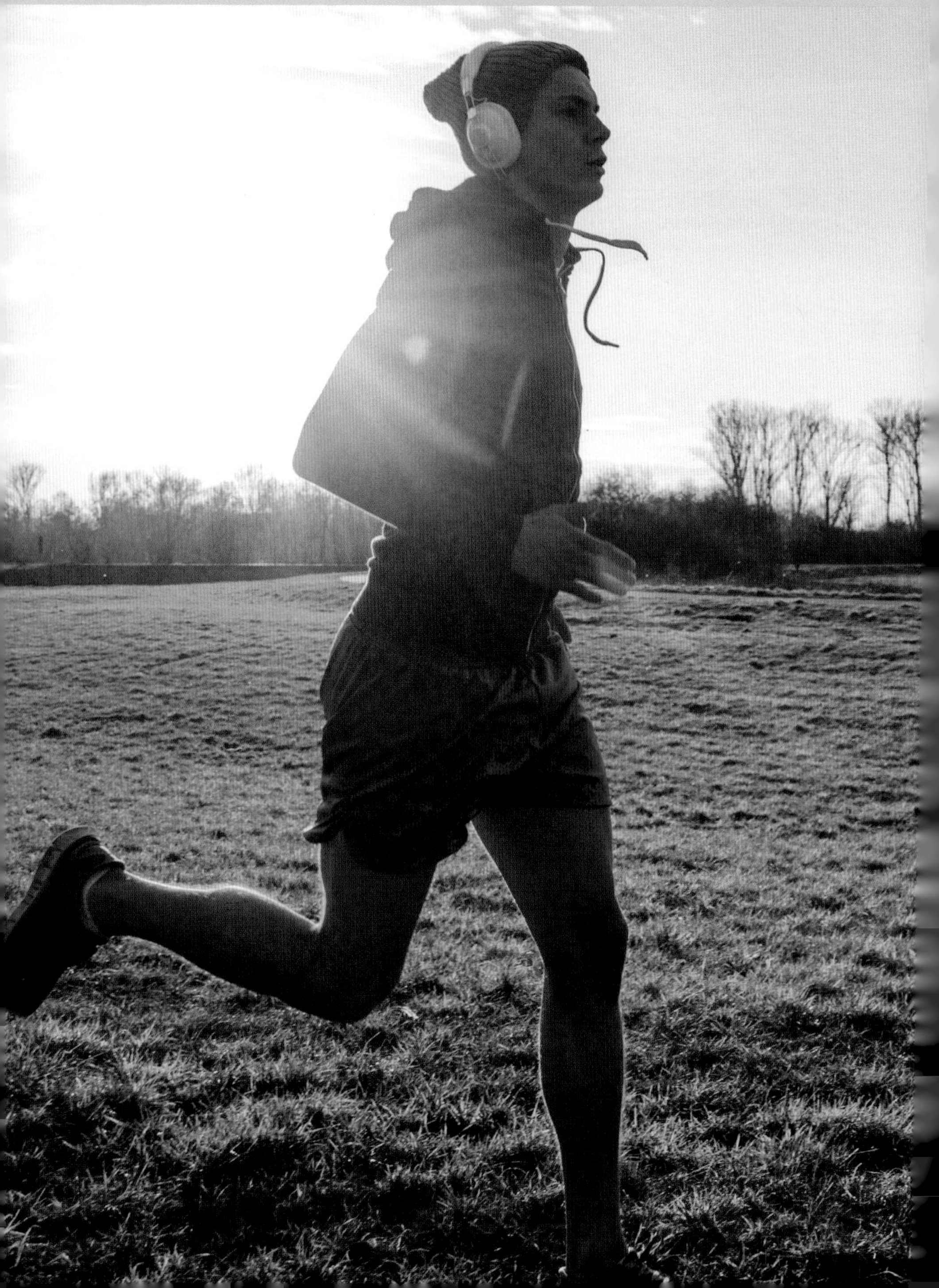

Mat Pilates exercises for runners

In this section of the book you will find a series of mat Pilates exercises, together with easy-to-follow instructions and photographs to guide you. Each exercise is graded as beginner, intermediate or advanced, and nearly all have options to modify or progress, so that you can choose to work at whichever level suits you best.

It's important to note that just because an exercise looks or feels 'easy', it doesn't mean that it isn't worth doing. All the exercises are in this book because they will help you to improve your running and stay injury-free. Too often we jump to the more challenging exercises in the hope that they will accelerate improvements – it doesn't work like that. So don't start with the advanced exercises before you have performed and understood the exercises for beginners.

At the end of this section you will find suggestions for 10–15 minute workouts that you can easily fit into your daily routine. Or you could even include them in your post-run cool down. These routines will also be graded into beginner, intermediate and advanced categories to suit your individual needs. Once you get to know the exercises, you'll be able to choose which ones are suitable for your needs and make up your own routine.

Musculoskeletal problems

If you have back, knee, hip or other musculoskeletal problems, please consult a medical practitioner before attempting any of these exercises. While Pilates improves core strength and so in many cases can alleviate back problems, it is important that you take it easy and read the instructions before attempting any of the exercises. Please take professional advice if you're in any doubt about the suitability of the movements you're performing in relation to any problem you may have. Many physiotherapists, sports therapists, osteopaths, chiropractors and GPs recommend Pilates – please make sure that if you're under the care of any of the above practitioners, you take their advice.

Before some of the exercises I have also noted certain cautions that may need to be considered. These apply to any specific problems you may have, and where it might be advisable to either adapt the exercise or omit it altogether. Again, if in doubt, please take advice from a medical practitioner or specialist.

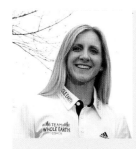

CASE STUDY: LIZ YELLING

Double Olympian and Commonwealth medallist Liz Yelling is a world class marathoner and respected female running coach (www. yellingperformance.com). Practising Pilates was an integral and important part of her own running training.

Pilates helped me focus on key areas of stability and conditioning that are important (but often neglected) by marathoners. It helped me hold some long periods of training together and improved the strength of my training foundation. During hard periods of training I was running 12 to 13 times a week and so having a robust body was very important to tolerate that workload. Pilates also helped in racing, particularly at the end of races when I needed my core to be strong and my form and posture to be maintained. Over the years, and as my running improved, I was constantly seeking out ways to improve and refine my performance and this often meant searching for ways to avoid injury! Pilates certainly helped – although when I first started doing it, it was more 'strength and conditioning' and could be quite a tough workout. As I grew to understand Pilates the focus certainly shifted towards focused, controlled movements. Now, with 3 children, I still regularly run, do low key events and particularly enjoy running on the trails. Although I'm no longer competing, looking after my body is still really important and I do make time for a weekly conditioning workout – usually done pushing my twin boys! This includes a variety of Pilates exercises - my favourite is the Table Top exercise with leg and arm extensions that really catch your abs out! It must be that feeling of the burn!

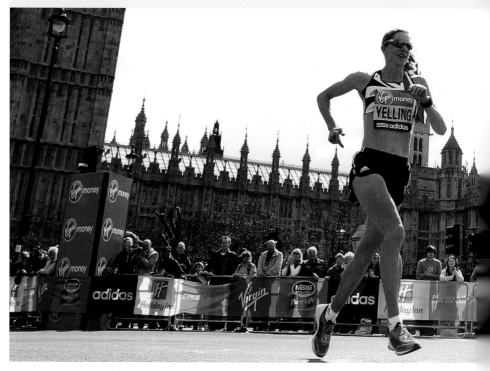

Liz Yelling passes Westminster during the Virgin London Marathon, April 2012

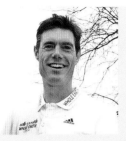

CASE STUDY: MARTIN YELLING

Martin Yelling is an endurance athlete and sports coach (www.yellingperformance.com). He is the joint host and founder of the UK's number one running podcast Marathon Talk (www.marathontalk.com). He is also the co-founder of Bournemouth Marathon Festival.

Pilates is really good for runners to help improve their overall body strength, control and conditioning. I think it's easy to get hooked on more and more miles, times and distance. Focusing on a strong foundation helps your body tolerate the training, recover and maintain consistency. It can also help with flexibility and range of motion. This is really important for holding form, technique and relaxation. Pilates is really important to me now. I prolapsed a disc in my lower back and it reinforced the need for me to pick up on the frequently neglected but very important aspects of looking after your body – and your back in particular. Now I go to a weekly local Pilates class with a group of friends and do short bouts of Pilates when I'm out running!

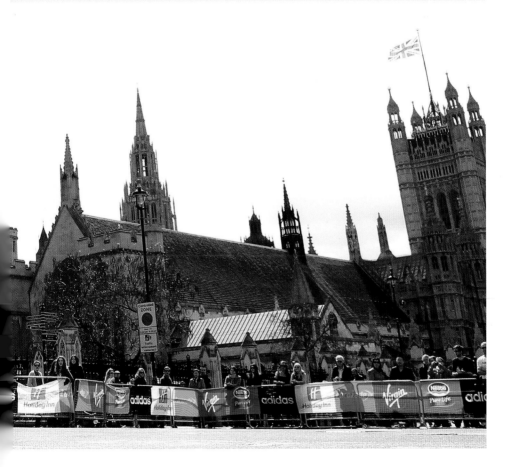

WARM UP

If you are performing these exercises after a run then you probably don't need to warm up – although the spinal Roll Down is a great post-run mobilizer and stretch for the spine and hamstrings and a very popular exercise with runners.

The warm up helps you to become centred, to grow aware of your body alignment and to start the lengthening process that the exercises encourage and require. It also promotes blood flow, joint mobility and enhances concentration. I've also included some exercises to improve balance and strengthen feet, both of which are integral to becoming a stronger runner.

You might like to perform your warm up in front of a long mirror so that you can keep an eye on your posture. If you're like most of my clients who don't want to look at themselves while they exercise, then you will think this is a dreadful idea, but I can't emphasize enough how useful this can be.

> I must be right. Never an aspirin. Never injured a day in my life. The whole country, the whole world, should be doing my exercises. They'd be happier.
>
> Joseph Pilates

Note: *if you have jumped straight to this warm up without reading Chapter 4 on postural alignment, please read it now so that you know and understand what all the terms used in the following exercises mean.*

Method

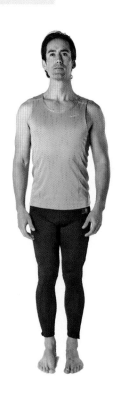

- Stand tall, shoulders stabilized, arms relaxed at your sides.
- Imagine the helium balloons are attached to the top of your head and lifting you upwards (page 30).
- Lengthen through the spine and don't forget to include your neck.
- Fix your gaze on something ahead of you.
- Perform a few pelvic tilts and find your neutral spine (page 28).
- Engage your abdominal/pelvic floor muscles.
- Breathe in through your nose and into your rib cage.
- Breathe out through your mouth.
- Repeat the breathing a couple more times and be aware of any muscular tensions in your body – try to consciously relax and let the breathing focus your attention.

Neck

- Keep the lengthening through your neck.
- Now drop your right ear to your right shoulder, gently stretching out the other side of your neck and upper back muscles.

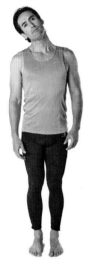

- Lift your head slowly back up to centre – repeat 4 times to the right shoulder.
- Perform the exercise to your left 4 times.
- Now drop your chin down on to your chest.
- Gently rotate your neck to your right shoulder but don't take your neck beyond your shoulder.

- Gently rotate to the other side – let the weight of your head carry it slowly from side to side.

- Repeat 2 more times either side, then come back to centre and lift up your head, lengthening through your neck and spine once again.

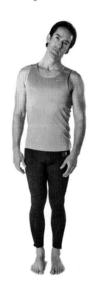

Shoulders

- Rotate your shoulders gently forwards 4 times.

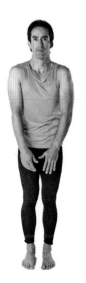

- Rotate your shoulders gently backwards 4 times.
- Lift your shoulders up around your ears.

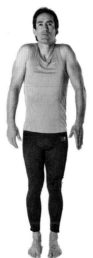

- Take them back, opening out your chest as you slide your shoulder blades down into your back pockets.
- Repeat 2 times.

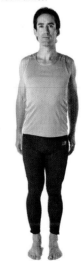

Spinal rotation

- Lengthen through the spine.
- Take your right hand and hold your left forearm near the elbow.
- Rotate your left arm to take hold of your right forearm near the elbow.
- Engage your abdominal/pelvic floor muscles.
- Breathe in to prepare.
- Breathe out and rotate your torso to the right, taking your head and neck with you.

- Concentrate on keeping your pelvis facing forwards as you rotate – it doesn't move with you, it needs to remain stable.
- Keep your shoulders relaxed and down.

- Breathe in and return to centre.
- Breathe out and rotate to the left.
- Breathe in and return to centre
- Repeat 3 times either side.

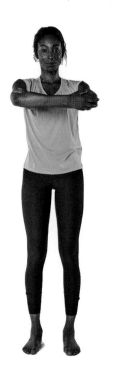

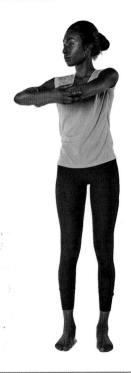

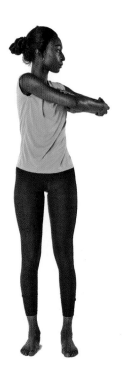

Lateral flexion (side bending)

- Standing tall again in neutral position (page 28), engage your abdominal/pelvic floor muscles.
- Breathe in to prepare.
- Breathe out and slide your right hand down the side of your right leg, lengthening your fingers as you do so.
- Hold the position.
- Breathe in.
- Imagine you are standing between two panes of glass, so your neck or chin aren't jutting forwards; you will be aligned with your whole body in the same plane.
- Breathe out and return to an upright position, lengthening through the spine as you do so and checking that your abdominal muscles are still engaged.
- Repeat on the other side.

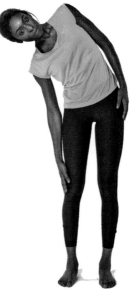
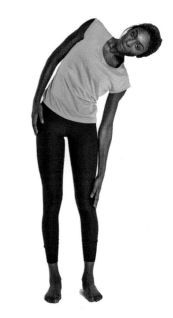

Knee, hip mobility and balance

- Standing tall, lengthen through your spine.
- Take your hands on to your hips but keep your shoulders relaxed.
- Engage your abdominal/pelvic floor muscles.
- Breathe naturally for this part of the warm up because it's more dynamic than the previous movements.
- Lift your knee up in front of you.

Try not to collapse in your centre and keep your gaze fixed ahead of you, still lengthening through the spine.
Take your leg back down to the floor.
Repeat 4 times on both sides.
Make sure the knee and foot are aligned. Imagine a vertical line through your knee to your foot, so that it is raised and aligned directly in front of you, not slightly to the side or crossing the centre of your body. If you look at your knee it should be in line with your second or third toe. Again, if you can stand in front of a mirror for this exercise it will help you with the placement.

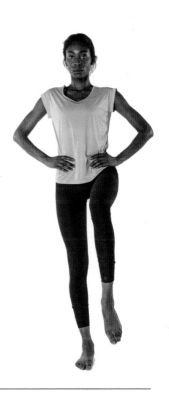

Hip opener and balance

- Stand tall, lengthening through the spine in neutral position (page 28), abdominal muscles engaged, hands on your hips, shoulders relaxed.
- Breathe naturally.
- Lift your right knee up in front of you.

- Open your hip to the side, taking your leg/knee with you but keeping your pelvis stable. Don't let the pelvis swing back.
- Bring the right leg back to centre and lower to the floor.
- Repeat 4 times and then change sides.

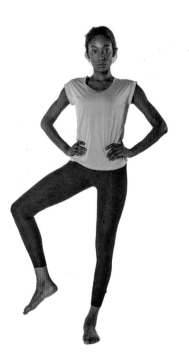 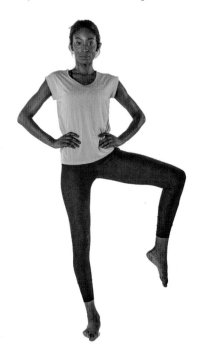

> Many injuries to the ankle and knees arise because of poor balance. If you have previously sprained your ankle, the proprioceptors (joint position sensors) will not be as efficient at detecting where your ankle is in space, so other structures in the lower extremity take the strain when you are running on uneven ground, or even on a pavement with a slight camber. Pilates can improve proprioception throughout the body, which will reduce unnecessary strain on joints, therefore preventing injury.
>
> Jane Kaushal, osteopath and runner

ROLL DOWN

Running benefits

This is a wonderful, relaxing exercise that can be used as a warm up. It is also excellent as a cool down and stretch after a run, or even mid-run should you have an achy back, tired glutes or tight hamstrings. It improves spinal mobility, allowing the spinal discs to expand, and encourages flexibility of the back and hamstrings. You might like to stick to the basic Roll Down exercise or add in the progressions for a deeper stretch.

Note: if you have serious lower back problems, please modify (page 54).

Method

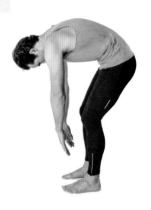

- Stand tall with shoulders relaxed and in neutral spine.
- Engage your abdominal/pelvic floor muscles.
- Keep your knees soft and very slightly bent.
- Breathe in to your rib cage to prepare.
- Breathe out as you bring your chin towards your chest.
- Slowly begin to roll yourself down towards the floor.
- Stop when you come to a comfortable point of tension.

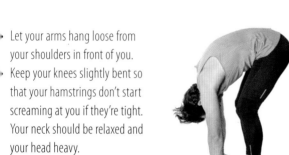

- Let your arms hang loose from your shoulders in front of you.
- Keep your knees slightly bent so that your hamstrings don't start screaming at you if they're tight. Your neck should be relaxed and your head heavy.

Imagine you are a rag doll as you gently 'hang', letting everything relax.

Breathe naturally and hold the 'rag doll' position for a few seconds. Breathe in to your rib cage. Breathe out and, making sure your abdominal/pelvic floor muscles are engaged to protect your spine, start to uncurl your body vertebrae by vertebrae, slowly building up your spine, strong, straight and tall.

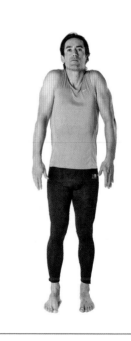

- As you reach the top, keep your gaze down to the last minute, then uncurl, lengthening through your spine.
- Breathe naturally and check your posture, lifting your shoulders up around your ears and sending your shoulder blades down into your back pockets again.

▶

- Check that you're still in neutral spine.
- Repeat the Roll Down 3 times in total – or as many times as you feel you want to.

Note
- Make sure you are bending through your spine and not your hips.
- Keep the weight evenly distributed through both feet; don't lean.

> I love doing the Roll Down. I find something very relaxing about being upside down and feeling the blood rush to my head as the spine stretches out. Plus it's my weekly opportunity to inspect what is going on with my toenails!
>
> Tania Baldwin-Pask, trail runner

Modify
- If you have lower back problems, place the palms of your hands on to your thighs. Slide them down your legs as you roll down, supporting your back in the process. If you feel any discomfort at all, stop.

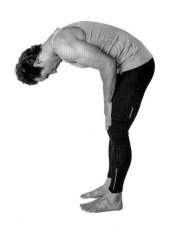

Progress
- For a deeper stretch, when you're in the 'rag doll' position, take the palms of your hands on to your opposite elbows and move your weight gently on to the balls of your feet. But take care you don't overbalance.
- Increasing the stretch further, in the roll down position, bend your right knee gently so that you get a stretch on the left side.
- Bring your right knee back and bend your left knee.
- Alternate between the two, keeping your feet on the ground, just easing and lengthening the muscles.

- Repeat 6 times then come to a standstill.
- Engage your abdominal/pelvic floor muscles.
- Breathe in.
- Breathe out and start to uncurl once again. Take you time and be aware of your alignment.

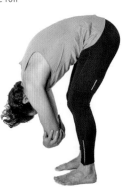
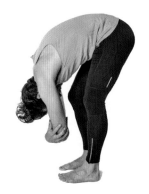

BALANCE

Running benefits

Balance is an important part of any running technique. As we age, our ability to balance declines, so it's important to practise. To balance well we need to have good coordination, strong ankles and feet (for foot strengthening exercises, see page 57). Balance exercises help the brain to recognize and cope with changes in terrain, and also help concentration. You might find that as you practise these exercises you discover that your balance is better on one side of the body than the other – we all have a dominant side.

Try to incorporate some kind of balance exercise into your everyday life – maybe stand on one leg while you're waiting for the kettle to boil, brushing your teeth in the morning or waiting at the school gates.

Method

Stand tall, lengthening through the spine in neutral spine position. Engage your abdominal/pelvic floor muscles.

Fix your gaze and concentrate on something ahead of you to help you balance.

Slowly lift your right knee directly in front of you a little way. Hold your balance, standing on one leg in this position for 30 seconds.

- Try not to hold your breath – breathe naturally.
- Lower the leg and change sides, repeating the balance for another 30 seconds.
- Return to the first side, raise your leg and find your balance, engage your abdominals and lengthen through the spine again.

- Breathe in and lift both arms up to the side and above your head.
- Breathe out and lower them to the sides of your body.
- Repeat the arm sequence once more, still standing on one leg.
- Change sides and repeat.

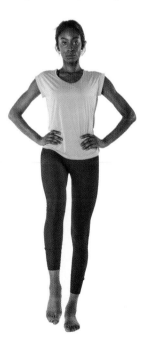
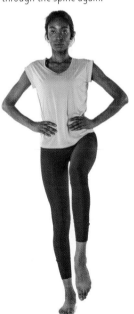
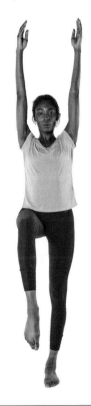

▶

Note

- During the exercises, if you find that you wobble a lot, hold on to something to begin with. Or touch the floor with your toe before taking the foot away and balancing. Each time you wobble, return your toe back to the floor for a second.

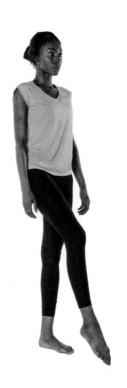

I've also taken it upon myself to try core-strengthening exercises of every conceivable description and difficulty. I've worked on my posture. I've tried to correct an instinctive, constant lean to the left, borne of being blind in one eye. And I've instigated several regimes of varying lunacy to try to improve my stability – once, every evening for a month, I cleaned my teeth standing on one leg with my eyes closed. All in a bid to lessen the chances of sustaining a running injury, and having to take time off.

Vassos Alexander, sports broadcaster and author of Don't Stop Me Now – 26.2 tales of a runner's obsession

- Take it slowly, and if you're holding on to something, every now and again let go; you'll find that your body will eventually get the message and your balance will improve. If you do these exercises in front of a mirror, you can make sure that your pelvis stays level and doesn't tilt to one side as you lift your leg, which could be a sign of gluteal weakness (see page 125 for the Shoulder Bridge exercise, which strengthens the glutes).
- Balance exercises are also good for all lower limb injuries (page 183).

Progress

- If you're confident with your ability to balance, try the exercise with your eyes closed.
- Please make sure that you don't fall!
- Keep the leg low to start with; touch the floor with your toe to get started.
- Hold for a few seconds and then increase the amount of time you keep your eyes closed.
- This can be challenging and demonstrates how important our visual sense is to maintaining balance.

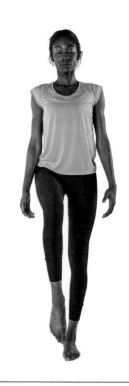

FOOT EXERCISES

Running benefits

When planning a regular cross-training routine, foot strengthening and stretching exercises are probably not one of the first things you think to include. But they are vital for strong running and are often neglected. At the risk of stating the obvious, your feet take a huge amount of impact when you run and also play a large part in stabilization. I include these exercises in all of my Pilates classes. Not only will they strengthen your feet, but also the muscles, ligaments and tendons attached.

Plantar fasciitis and Achilles tendonitis are common running injuries that can be prevented (pages 184 and 187). I also include an Ankle Mobility and foot stretch exercise on page 107, but the following exercises can be practised whenever you get the opportunity and preferably in bare feet.

ACHILLES AND CALF MUSCLE STRENGTHENER

Method

- Stand tall, lengthening through the spine.
- Slowly begin to pedal up and down on the balls of your feet — come right up, nearly on to your toes.
- Repeat 10 times in total.
- Now come up on to the balls of both feet together and balance. Hold the position for the count of 4.

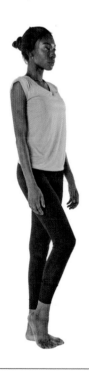
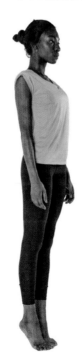

- Lower both heels back down to the mat as slowly as you can.
- Repeat 4 times, keeping the movement slow and controlled.
- Perform 10 heel lifts fast — feel those calf muscles working!

BRAIN GYM FOR FEET AND BALANCE

This simple exercise will not only stretch and strengthen your feet but also challenge your stability and coordination.

Method

- Stand tall, lengthening through the spine.
- Rise up on to the ball of your right foot only.

- Now come up on to the ball of your left foot.
- Take your right heel slowly down to the floor.

- Take your left heel down.
- Rise up on to the ball of your right foot and follow it with your left.
- Repeat 5 times in total and then change sides, starting on the left.

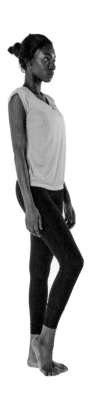
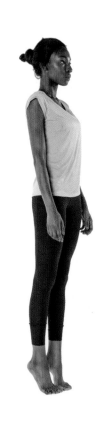
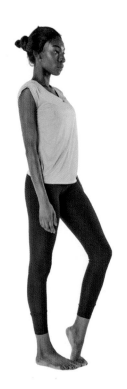

HEEL AND TOE WALKS

Method

- Stand tall, lengthening through the spine.
- Walk forwards on your toes for 10 steps.
- Walk backwards on your heels for 10 steps.

- Repeat the sequence several times. This can also be performed in trainers as part of your dynamic warm up before a run.

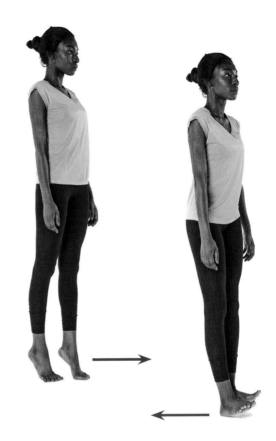

CASE STUDY

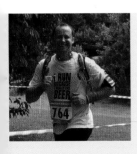

Phil Pask has run 30+ half-marathons, runs 2–3 times a week and attends a weekly Pilates class.

Pilates has improved all aspects of my posture and running, with the knock-on benefit of less pulling on my back which used to occur on the longer runs and half marathons. I hardly get any lower back tension any more thanks to this. It has helped improve my core strength and even though I still need to work on it, it really helps me with my hill running. I use my arms and my whole body better. When I look back on my pre-Pilates running I think I was really only using my lower body and legs. By having better posture I run with more efficiency – more of my energy actually goes into propelling me than my 'non-upright' running was doing. Before Pilates, after a half marathon I wouldn't want to move for the rest of the day, now I can live a useful 'chore-filled' life after only a short period of stretching and relaxing. I do make my post-run stretches include some of the Pilates exercises, mainly the Roll Down which is my favourite and is really relaxing and feels as though it helps me all over – back, legs, shoulders.

BACK SERIES

SWAN DIVE (ALL LEVELS)

Running benefits

The Swan Dive exercise strengthens the mid/upper back and abdominal muscles. Those rounded, forward-slumped shoulders that surface when you're beginning to feel tired during a run can mean that the mobility of this area starts to be restricted. Hunched running posture can hamper your breathing as well. This exercise will help open out the chest area and strengthen the middle of your back (see thoracic spine, page 27), so that when tiredness hits, your posture and your running don't suffer.

Method

- Lie down on your front.
- Place a block or small cushion under your forehead – this is to keep your neck and spine aligned.
- Bend your arms so that your elbows are level with your shoulders and resting on the floor.
- Take your legs hip distance apart with your toes slightly turned in.

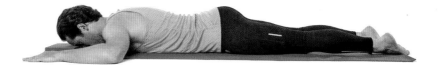

- Engage your abdominal/pelvic floor muscles.
- Breathe in to your rib cage to prepare.
- Breathe out as you gently lift your head, your chest, your arms and elbows off the floor.
- Breathe in at the top.

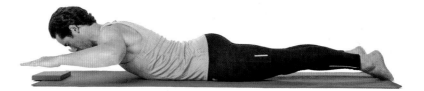

- Breathe out as you lower yourself slowly back to the floor.
- Repeat 8 times in total.

Note

- Keep your neck and spine aligned, lengthening through your neck as you raise your head.
- Try to keep the movement flowing and not jerky.
- Your legs and glutes will want to help you; try your best to keep them relaxed and immobile.
- Concentrate on your breathing and stay centred, pulling your abdomen up off the floor and engaging it throughout the exercise.
- If you get cramp in your foot, just curl your toes underneath and hopefully that will relieve the discomfort.

When you are doing as I am now, building up my running miles and times, or when you are in training for a race there is nothing better than working on the core muscles and feeling your strength improving and supporting you as you run. Pilates is irreplaceable. You can hone in on tension spots and really stretch out any problem areas while at the same time maintaining and improving your strength and posture.

Valerie Dornbach, 5k, 10k and half marathon runner

Modify

- Perform fewer repetitions.
- Raise your chest up with forearms still on the floor instead of lifting your arms.
- Keep the arms light. Try not to push down hard on the floor as you want your back muscles to work.

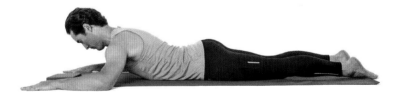

Follow with a Cat Stretch (page 82) to lengthen your spine in the opposite direction.

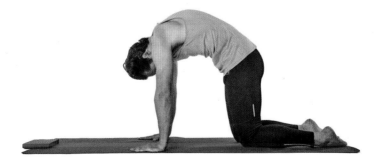

SUPERMAN (ALL LEVELS)

Running benefits

This is an excellent exercise for runners because it trains you to keep your torso stable while you move your arms and legs, which is exactly what we want to have happen when we run. It encourages good coordination and strengthens and lengthens the spinal extensor (erector spinae) muscles which support the spine, improving running posture while building stability in the core and shoulder muscles.

Note: if you find it uncomfortable to kneel on the floor or you have problems with your knees, either pad the knee area with a towel or choose the Swimming exercise on page 66 instead.

Method

- Start on all fours, knees directly under hips, arms under your shoulders.
- Keep your neck and spine aligned, with your eyes focused on the floor.

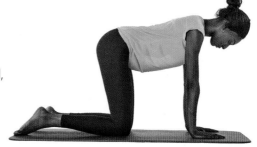

- Engage your abdominal/pelvic floor muscles.
- Breathe in to prepare.
- Breathe out through your mouth and slowly slide your left foot directly behind you on the floor, toes pointed, while simultaneously extending your right arm up in front of you.

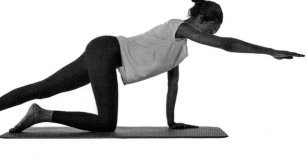

- When your leg is completely extended behind you, lift it to hip height and raise your arm, lengthened also, level with your ear.
- Balance and hold that position.

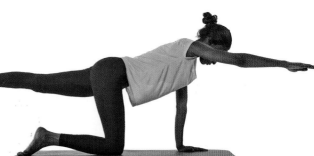

- Breathe in to your rib cage.
- Breathe out as you simultaneously lower both your arm and leg, with control, back down to the floor.
- Repeat on the other side.
- Repeat up to 10 times (5 each side).
- After you've completed this exercise, come into the Extended Child's Pose (page 85) so that any tensions are released. While in the Extended Child's Pose, stretch your arms ahead of you and rotate your wrists. Stay in that position for about 20 seconds. Then take your arms round by your sides to relieve any tension in your shoulders.

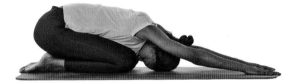

Note

- Be aware of your pelvis – is it dropping down on one side or shifting outwards as you lift your leg up to hip height?
- Aim to keep your torso as stable as possible, so be aware of your pelvis – imagine you are balancing a tray of full champagne glasses on your back.
- Keep the exercise flowing, concentrate on your breathing and keep centred.

Modify

- If you find the balancing a challenge, leave the arms out to begin with and concentrate purely on the legs. Alternate the legs 8 times in total.
- When you feel confident that you can keep your pelvis aligned and torso stable, you can introduce the arms.

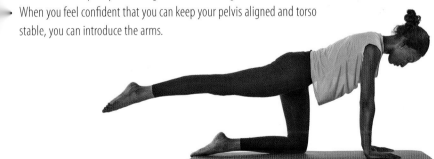

DART WITH TRICEP LIFTS (ALL LEVELS)

Running benefits
This exercise is primarily a back strengthener and mobilizer with the added bonus of some arm and shoulder work. It also encourages good running posture by extending the spine. Strengthening the triceps (back of arms) and shoulders will prevent the arms from becoming tired while running. This exercise will give you more strength and power to propel yourself forwards.

Method
- Lie on your front, arms down by your sides, palms turned up.
- Bring your big toes together and let your heels flop open to relax your legs.

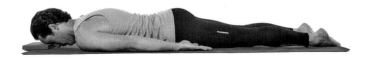

- Engage your abdominal/pelvic floor muscles.
- Breathe in to prepare.
- As you breathe out, lift your head, chest and arms up off the floor.

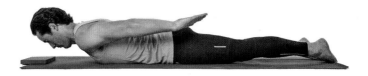

- Using short out breaths, pulse your arms upwards from the shoulders for the count of 10 pulses.

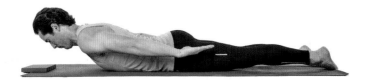

- On completion of the 10 pulses, hold the position.
- Breathe in to your rib cage again.
- Breathe out through your mouth as you return your chest and arms back to the floor.
- Repeat up to 8 times in total.

- Follow with a Cat Stretch (page 82) to lengthen your spine in the opposite direction.

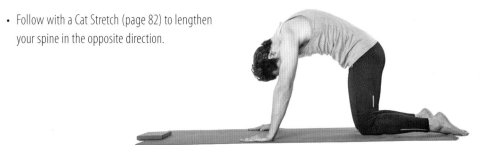

Note

- Make sure you are keeping your neck and spine aligned – look down, rather than tilting your head upwards.
- Remember to lengthen the neck – it sometimes gets forgotten!

- Avoid tensing your shoulders, and keep your abdominal muscles engaged throughout.
- Concentrate on your breathing to help the exercise flow.

Progress

- Increase the repetitions.
- Use hand weights. But make sure that if you do, you keep your neck lengthened and your legs relaxed. Don't let the hand weights alter the alignment of your body.

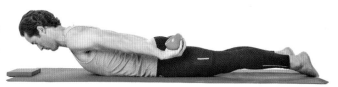

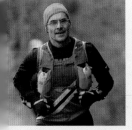

CASE STUDY

Steve Carroll from Frome is an ultra marathon runner and UK Athletics qualified coach. In 2015 alone he ran five marathons, five 50k races and a 50-mile race, all in the space of 10 months. In 2016 he ran the 86-mile Wessex Ridgeway.

As I wanted to run further in 2016 I started to think about supplementary training that would help my running. A friend suggested a Pilates class that she attended so I thought I would give it a go. I have been going weekly ever since. The sessions are challenging and I've definitely noticed over the months that I am getting stronger/more controlled through the exercises. I recently ran the Imber Ultra for the third consecutive year and knocked 19 minutes off my time from the year before and in the last two months have trimmed two minutes off my 10k PB, and while I can't directly attribute all of the improvements to Pilates I am sure is responsible for some. Also, being a UK Athletics qualified coach I am aware of the importance of good running form/posture. I definitely feel that the Pilates is helping with my running and that there much value in adding Pilates to ultra marathon training.

SWIMMING INTO BACK EXTENSION (ALL LEVELS)

Running benefits
Just like the Superman exercise (page 62), Swimming encourages torso and spinal stability while moving the arms and legs. Your core muscles have to constantly stabilize your pelvis when running, even more so on uneven trail routes. This exercise teaches the core muscles to work together and provide enough strength for us to stay upright, stable and strong when running. It also, like most Pilates exercises, lengthens the back, arm and leg muscles, especially those hip flexors and hamstrings which are notorious for becoming tight.

Method
- Lie on your front with your arms above your head as if you're about to dive into a swimming pool.

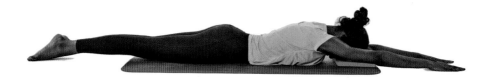

- Engage your abdominal/pelvic floor muscles. Pull your abdominal muscles in, lifting up off the floor. Try to keep them there.
- Breathe in to prepare.
- Breathe out, raise and lengthen both your arms and legs, keeping them parallel to the floor.

- Lift your head, keeping your neck and spine aligned.
- Breathe in for 5 counts while you gently pulse your arms and legs up and down dynamically as if paddling/swimming.

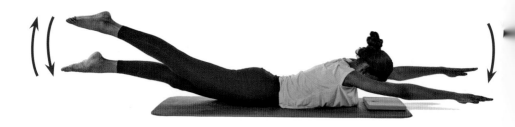

- Breathe out through your mouth for 5 counts, still paddling your arms and legs.
- Complete 4 sets of 10 paddles and then relax for a moment before continuing on to the Back Extension.

Back Extension

- Breathe in to prepare.
- Breathe out.
- Lift and extend both arms, both legs and your head.
- Hold for 5 seconds but remember to breathe naturally.

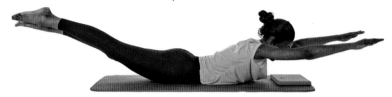

- Breathe in to your rib cage again.
- Breathe out as you lower yourself back to the ground.
- Repeat 4 times in total and then come into the Cat Stretch (page 82) followed by the Extended Child's Pose (page 85).

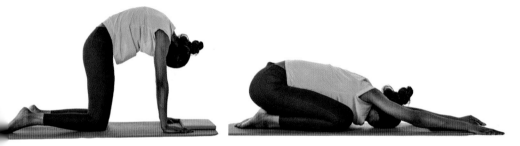

Note

- Keep your abdominal muscles lifted off the floor and engaged.
- Make sure you don't overextend your back.
- Concentrate and keep focused on your breathing and alignment.

Modify

To make the exercise easier, perform fewer repetitions or just raise the opposite arm to leg as in the Superman exercise (page 62).

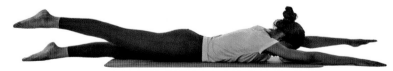

Progress

Increase the repetitions.

Use ankle weights – but if you do, make sure you can keep your body aligned. Don't let the ankle weights change the position of your body.

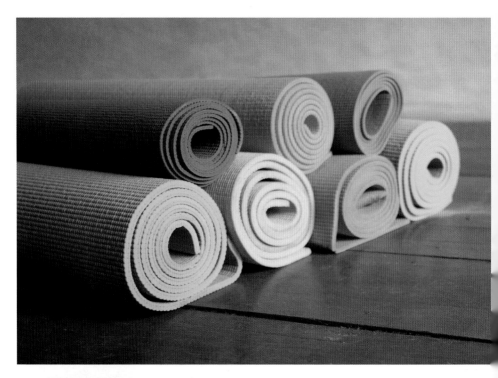

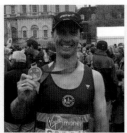

CASE STUDY

Neil King describes himself as a decent club runner who loves the many aspects of running – improved fitness, general well-being, beautiful scenery, good company and the challenge of battling with the terrain and the elements.

I've been running for four and a half years. After entering the Great North Run I caught the bug and have been racing ever since. I've completed seven road marathons, including a 3hr 1 min London Marathon at the age of 45. I now prefer trail off-road running and have completed 11 races between marathon and ultra marathon distances. I prefer the challenge of long-distance running and will be taking part in a 55-mile race in the next couple of weeks. I started Pilates about five years ago. I took it up as I'm a self-employed gardener and was experiencing back pain and sciatica. Pilates has significantly reduced the back pain, with much fewer episodes of sciatica, and it considerably improved my running ability. Over long-distance races there is the tendency to lose form and slump as fatigue sets in. Pilates and additional core training helps to keep correct upright posture and my stamina has improved. In addition, recovery post-race has been much quicker. I think the Pilates session as a whole though rather than any specific exercise provides the benefits. Post-race the stretching elements, such as Cobra stretch and Down Dog, help the most. Core exercises such as Swimming, Shoulder Bridge and Plank are very beneficial and provide me with a good basis for physical labour, every day well-being and endurance training.

LEG PULL FRONT/PLANK (INTERMEDIATE/ADVANCED)

Running benefits

This is a version of the well-known Plank exercise which encourages pelvic and shoulder stabilization while strengthening all the core muscles and of course your arms. Not only that, but it also stretches the front of the hips and calf muscles. Leg Pull exercises are very powerful and will improve your running endurance, stability and power – other exercises are the Side Plank/Leg Pull (page 96) and Reverse Plank / Leg Pull (page 134).

Note: if you have weak wrists, a shoulder injury or find your abdominal muscles aren't quite strong enough to perform this exercise yet, modify and adapt accordingly.

Method

- Start the exercise on your hands and knees.
- Make sure your hands are aligned under your shoulders.
- Slide one leg directly behind you and come on to the ball of the foot.

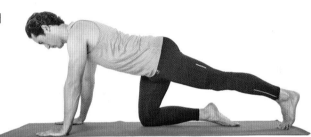

- Repeat on the other side until you are in the Leg Pull position.

Engage your abdominal muscles/ pelvic floor muscles.
Breathe in to prepare.

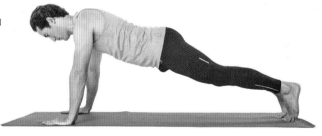

Breathe out and lift one leg off the floor, at the same time pushing the heel of the other foot down towards the floor.
Breathe in and hold.
Breathe out and lower the leg back down into the start position.
Repeat on the other side.
Repeat the leg movement, alternating 6 times.

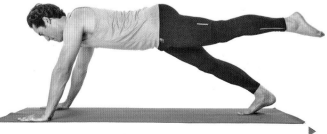

▶

- At the end of the exercise come into the Extended Child's Pose.

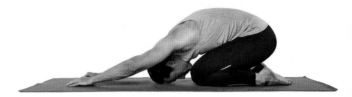

Note

- Once in the Leg Pull position, there should be a straight line from your feet to your head.
- Keep in this neutral spine position.
- Make sure your back doesn't sag or your bottom lift up – remember you are a plank!

- Keep your abdominal muscles activated throughout.
- Focus on your breathing as it will help with concentration.

Modify 1 (beginner)

- Lie on your front and come up on to your forearms – elbows directly below your shoulders.

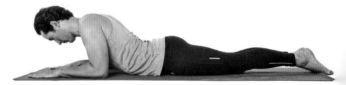

- Engage your abdominal/pelvic floor muscles.
- Breathe in to prepare.
- Breathe out as you lift your pelvis a little way and come on to your knees, feeling your abdominal muscles contract as you do so.

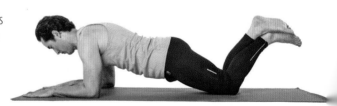

- Breathe in to your rib cage and then out through your mouth – continue using your lateral thoracic breathing to help you concentrate and stay put.
- Make sure you keep the neck and spine aligned and that your abdominal/pelvic floor muscles stay engaged.

- If you start to feel tension in your back, then stop, come down on to the floor, rest for a second or two and try again – you should feel the abdominal muscles working.
- Hold for up to 30 seconds – or longer if you can!

Modify 2 (intermediate)

- Lie on your front and come up on to your forearms — elbows placed directly below your shoulders.

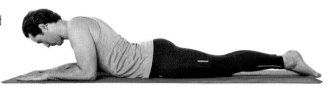

- Engage your abdominal/pelvic floor muscles.
- Breathe in to prepare.
- Breathe out and lift yourself up into a straight line and on to the balls of your feet.

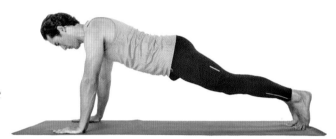

- Stabilize in that position and concentrate on breathing — in through your nose and into your rib cage and then out through your mouth, for a total of 5 breaths.
- Keep your legs lengthened and feet on the floor.
- Maintain your neck and spine alignment throughout — don't drop your head down or tilt it upwards.

I started running 14 years ago, but three years later I slipped two discs when I was picking something heavy up off the floor. Obviously I had to stop running and was referred to a consultant who told me I had a choice, either surgery, or because I was already fit, Pilates and physio. So I chose the latter. After about a year of practising Pilates I didn't need painkillers any more. A six-month scan showed that the discs had naturally gone back in. They'll always be weak but Pilates taught me so much – it made me look at my posture, how I was standing, sitting, and also made me aware of how to correctly pick heavy things up off the floor by engaging my core muscles. Three years ago, at the age of 55, I braved trying to run again. I missed it so much but was really scared of aggravating my back. I started with a beginners' group and slowly progressed to running 3- and 5-milers twice a week, which makes me very happy! And I know I couldn't do it without Pilates. It keeps my back in check. I'm also aware of my posture when I run, making sure that I am upright, I feel better when I'm lengthening through my spine rather than slouching. There's no doubt about it, Pilates has enabled me to run.

Janet Lee, recreational runner

ROTATIONAL CAT (ALL LEVELS)

Running benefits

The Rotational Cat exercise will strengthen your core muscles and challenge your balance. It will also increase flexibility throughout the whole of your back as it rotates your spine and will open out and stretch your chest muscles. The thoracic spine (page 27) can become stiff and rounded on a long run, and this exercise will encourage good posture and over time will prevent this from happening. This is also a great exercise for the day after a long run if you tend to suffer from post-run back ache; or if you sit slouched over a desk all day, you'll find the rotational movement of the exercise relieves the postural tension that this can cause.

Note: if it's uncomfortable to kneel on the floor, place a rolled-up towel underneath each knee for more comfort. If you have wrist or elbow problems you might want to omit this exercise.

Method

- Start the exercise on your hands and knees.
- Place your hands directly under your shoulders, knees under your hips.
- Keep your head and spine aligned.
- Engage your abdominal/pelvic floor muscles.
- Breathe in to prepare.
- Breathe out, take your right arm off the ground and thread it between your left arm and left leg.

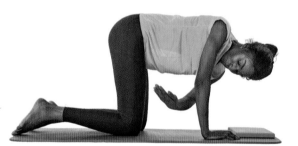

- Bend your left elbow.
- Lower your head and right shoulder down to the mat for a deeper rotation as long as you are comfortable to do so.
- Breathe in and hold the rotational stretch.

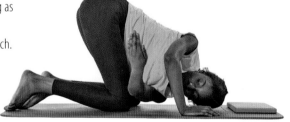

- Breathe out and rotate back the other way, taking your right arm up in the air, this time following it with your head and neck.
- Breathe in at the top as you hold the position.

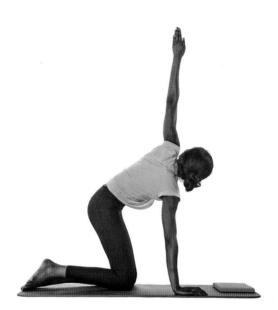

- Breathe out as you return to the mat.
- Continue rotating, keeping the exercise flowing from side to side.
- Repeat 6 times, and then come down into the Extended Child's pose (page 85) to give your wrist a rest before changing sides.

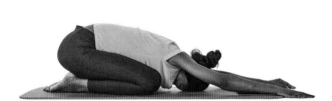

Note
- Don't force the rotation; only go as far as you are comfortable.
- Keep your abdominal muscles engaged throughout.
- Let the exercise flow and concentrate on your breathing.

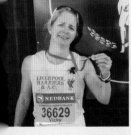

CASE STUDY

Vicky Unsworth, 34, from Liverpool, is a 2hr 28m London Marathon Championship runner. She has run 20 marathons.

I definitely think having a strong core helps me run better. I have very little time to do strength and conditioning but find doing a few Pilates exercises every day helps. When I get tired in a race and lose my form I always think about my core and try to run from it. It helps focus my mind somewhere else and helps me to hopefully run a bit quicker. For a few years I hit a bit of a plateau, then I had a baby. Pilates definitely helped during those times and I've now become faster in all distances. I think a lot of people just focus on running without doing anything else, when a strong body, good diet, lots of sleep and recovery all help to go into the mix of making us better runners.

THE SINGLE LEG KICK (BEGINNER)

Running benefits

This exercise will give your quads and hip flexors a good stretch. When you're running the hip flexors work hard repeatedly raising your leg: they contract and shorten each time. So if they become tight your pelvis can begin to tilt forwards and this can lead to back ache. The Single Leg Kick will also strengthen the glutes, hamstrings, upper arms and back. The glutes can often be a problem for runners, either because they're not firing properly or are weak – often the cause of lumbar and pelvic instability – as discussed in Chapter 3. If you want to increase your speed and run those hills comfortably, strengthen your glutes and hamstrings!

Note: if you have knee problems, please modify.

Method

- Lie on your front.
- Come on to your forearms, elbows sitting just below your shoulders.
- Make fists with your hands.

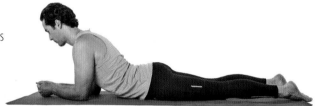

- Engage your abdominal/pelvic floor muscles.
- Breathe in to your rib cage to prepare.
- Breathe out and kick your heel towards your buttock, pulsing twice.

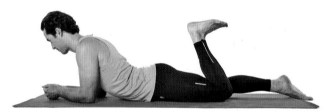

- Lengthen and extend the leg back out along the floor as you breathe in again.

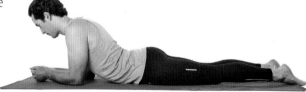

- Breathe out and repeat with your other leg, pulsing twice and then extending back along the floor as you breathe in.
- Repeat 8 times, alternating legs, and then come into the Cat Stretch (page 82).

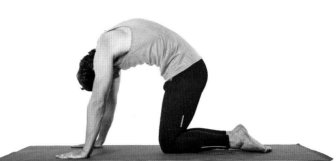

Note

- Make sure you keep your abdominal muscles engaged throughout the exercise.
- Be aware of any arching in your back and your general alignment.
- Concentrate on your breathing to help the exercise flow more easily.

Modify

- Be careful if you have knee problems: rather than kicking, keep the movement smooth and move the leg only in a comfortable range, don't pulse. Or omit the exercise altogether.

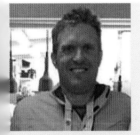

CASE STUDY

Paul Buckle from Suffolk likes a challenge, both mental and physical. So he runs ultra marathons – he's run 35 marathon-plus distance events including eight ultras. His maximum distance to date is 100 miles, and now he is training for the King Offas Dyke Ultra which is 186 miles. Paul enjoys doing consecutive day events, running trails, and he attends a Pilates class once a week.

My wife introduced me to Pilates. I joined an all-male class on a Wednesday evening about a year ago. At first I was skeptical about it but now I wouldn't be without it. I thought it wouldn't benefit me but how wrong I was! The studio is about three miles from my house and so I try to run to class and home again afterwards. My run home after a Pilates class is far more comfortable and effortless. I have often joked that I should do a class before my races. Not such a stupid idea though! I have been injury-free since starting Pilates, although I still have niggles and pains but most runners do. I have had no major injuries in the last year though. I believe my stamina has improved and my strength, both physical and mental – my core strength has definitely improved. Many of the events I take part in require the carrying of a rucksack, sometimes reasonably heavy. This takes its toll on my back, shoulders and arms. Pilates helps with this. Of course breathing is an important element of Pilates and this helps with longer distance runs.

THE DOUBLE LEG KICK (INTERMEDIATE/ADVANCED)

Running benefits

This exercise is a progression from the Single Leg Kick (page 74), so make sure you are comfortable with that exercise before attempting this one. The Double Leg Kick generates the same running benefits as the Single Leg Kick but is more challenging, strengthening the glutes, hip flexors and back muscles while stretching the front of the thighs and opening out the chest. It also challenges stability and improves coordination – everything a runner needs in an exercise!

Note: if you have knee problems, please modify.

Method

- Lie on your front.
- Turn your head to one side.
- Take both hands to your lower back and clasp them together.
- Let your elbows sink towards the floor at the side of your torso.
- Bring your extended legs together and point your toes.

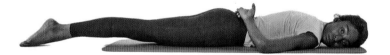

- Engage your abdominal/pelvic floor muscles.
- Breathe in to your rib cage to prepare.
- Breathe out as you bend your knees and kick both heels towards your buttocks, pulsing three times.
- Breathe in as you lengthen the legs back along the mat.

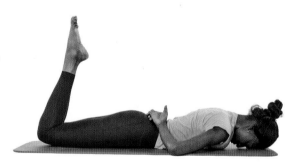

- Breathe out as you lift your chest off the floor, straightening your arms, hands still clasped along your back, simultaneously lifting your legs and lengthening them away from you.

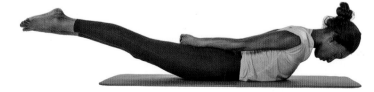

- Breathe in, lower the legs and your torso back down to the floor, turning your head to face the other direction.
- Breathe out and relax.
- Repeat 6 times in total, then come into an Extended Child's Pose.

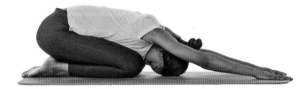

Note

- You may find it easier to breathe naturally to begin with and perform this exercise dynamically.
- Keep your legs lengthened together.
- Keep your hips glued to the mat as you kick your heels back.

Modify

- Be careful if you have knee problems: perform the exercise slowly within a comfortable range of movement. Or omit the exercise altogether.
- Perform Single Leg Kick (page 74).
- If your shoulders are stiff, leave your arms down by your sides and just perform the leg movements.

Progress

- Increase the repetitions.
- Reach your clasped hands further down your back and lift your torso higher.

Pilates has definitely had a positive impact on me since I started it two years ago, following the birth of my second daughter. Originally it was to strengthen my groin, but I've continued going to my weekly class because of the difference that I see in my posture and flexibility. Since training for a marathon, I've been convinced it has kept me injury-free, and the class has been a vital addition to my training programme. This was highlighted recently with a holiday that meant I did not do Pilates for three weeks in the middle of my marathon training. I picked up a leg injury and could not run for a week. It definitely makes a difference and I feel it when I miss a class.

Emma Hellewell ran her first (and last... so she says) London Marathon in April 2016

PUSH UP FROM STANDING (INTERMEDIATE/BEGINNER)

Running benefits

This can be a challenging exercise but an excellent arm (especially triceps) and pectoral (chest) strengthening exercise. It encourages good shoulder stability, core strength and spinal mobility. Over time this will improve your running posture, arm drive and stability. In addition this exercise will lengthen your hamstrings and quads.

Method

- Stand tall, lengthening through the spine into neutral spine position.
- Engage your abdominal/pelvic floor muscles.
- Breathe in to prepare.
- Breathe out and slowly roll down towards your mat (see Roll Down, page 53) with your legs straight until your hands reach or nearly reach the ground.

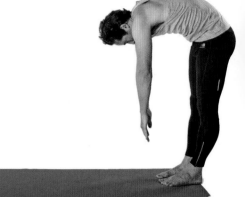

- Breathe in.
- Breathe out and walk your hands forwards, keeping your heels down and legs straight.

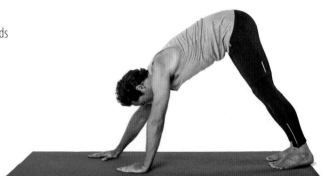

- Breathing naturally, come down into the Leg Pull Front/Plank position (page 69), hands aligned under your shoulders.

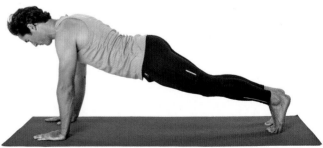

- Bend your knees down on to the floor.
- Cross your ankles and bring your heels up behind your buttocks.

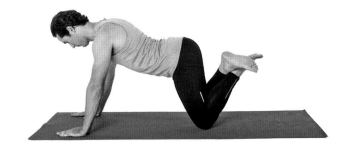

- Breathe in as you take your torso down to the mat.

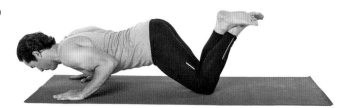

- Breathe out as you push up.
- Repeat 3 Push Ups in total.

- Breathe in and push your hips up towards the ceiling.
- Breathe out and walk your hands back towards your feet.
- Breathe in and hold the position.
- Breathe out and slowly uncurl back up to standing.
- Repeat up to 3 times.

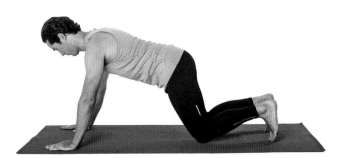

Modify

If you find this exercise too challenging, move your hands slightly wider than your shoulders before you perform the Push Up – this won't target the triceps quite so much but will still work those arm muscles. Keep the Push Up small until you feel stronger.

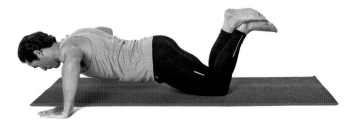

PUSH UP FROM STANDING (ADVANCED)

Note: if you have wrist, elbow or shoulder problems, take care. Modify the exercise (page 81) if you feel that you can't maintain the position.

Method
- Stand tall, lengthening through the spine into neutral spine position.
- Engage your abdominal/pelvic floor muscles.
- Breathe in to prepare.
- Breathe out and slowly roll down towards your mat (see Roll Down, page 53) with your legs straight until your hands reach or nearly reach the ground. If you have tight hamstrings, just go as far as you comfortably can.

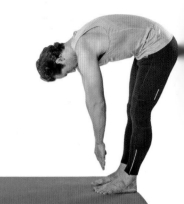

- Breathe in.
- Breathe out and walk your hands forwards, keeping your heels down on the floor, or as near to the floor as possible and legs straight.

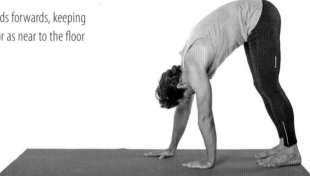

- Breathing naturally, come down into the Leg Pull Front/Plank position (page 69), hands aligned under your shoulders.

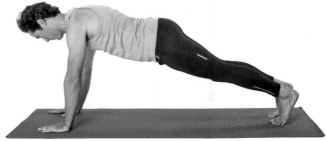

- Breathe in and lower yourself slowly towards the floor, keeping your elbows close to your ribs as they bend.

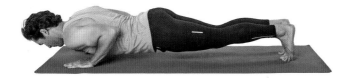

- Breathe out and push up back into the Plank position.

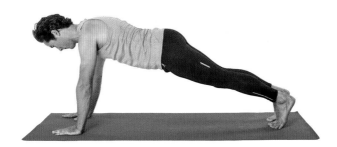

Repeat 3 Push Ups in total.
Breathe in and push your hips up towards the ceiling.
Breathe out and walk your hands back towards your feet.
Hold the position as you breathe in.
Breathe out and slowly uncurl back up to standing.
Repeat up to 6 times, each time performing 3 Push Ups.

Note

- Don't be tempted to move your hands forwards, keep them aligned under the shoulders.
- Try and stroke your ribs with your elbows as you lower yourself to the ground.
- Keep your abdominal muscles engaged throughout.
- Concentrate on your breathing and keep the movement slow and controlled.
- Maintain neutral spine throughout.

odify

Push Up from Standing (intermediate/beginner), page 78.
Perform fewer repetitions.
Keep the Push Up small until you feel stronger.

> A strong core and robust body is essential for any runner in order to train hard and reach potential. But in our everyday lives we can spend far too much time sitting down which shortens our hamstrings and weakens our glutes and core muscles. So we need an exercise system that targets these areas – Pilates does just that.
>
> Matt Whiting, former running coach to Phil Wicks, GB International athlete and 2hr 15mins marathon runner

CAT STRETCH (ALL LEVELS)

Running benefits

This is a wonderful yoga-based post-run (or any-time) stretch. It is also an excellent spinal mobilizer, especially if you have a tight lower back. You'll see that I've suggested performing this exercise as a relief stretch at the end of some of the previous exercises, especially in the Back Series: it's a good way of stretching the spine in the opposite direction to the way in which you've been working. The Cat Stretch also works the abdominal muscles.

Method

- Come on to all fours.
- Align your hands under your shoulders, your knees under your hips.

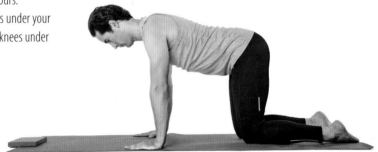

- Engage your abdominal/pelvic floor muscles.
- Breathe in to prepare.
- Breathe out as you arch your back up towards the ceiling, dropping your head and neck – like a cat hissing!

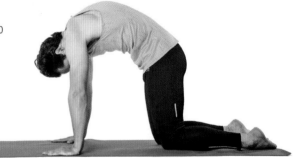

- Hold the stretch as you breathe in again.
- Breathe out and bring your spine back into neutral.
- Repeat 3 times or more.

Note
- You can hold the stretch for as long as you feel you need to.
- Breathe naturally and feel the muscles lengthening in your back as you do so.

CAT STRETCH INTO DOWN DOG

Running benefits

A great exercise to lengthen the hamstrings, calf muscles and Achilles tendons either post-run or during an exercise routine. It also strengthens the upper body and spine to encourage coordination – a great combination of yoga and Pilates.

Method

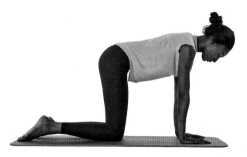 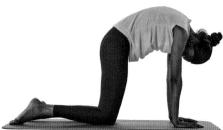

- Start on all fours in a neutral position.
- Make sure your arms are aligned under your shoulders, your knees under your hips.

- Engage your abdominal/pelvic floor muscles.
- Breathe in to prepare.
- Breathe out as you lengthen through your spine and arch into the Cat Stretch.

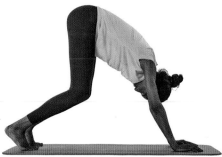 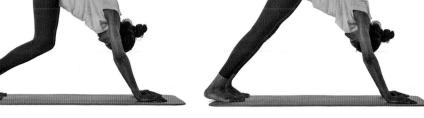

Curl your toes under, drop your head and lift your knees.
Breathe in as you send your spine up into the air, your tailbone towards the ceiling.

- Breathe out as you lengthen your calf muscles and gently ease your heels down on to the floor.
- Breathe in and hold the calf stretch.

▶

- Breathe out and come on to the balls of your feet, keeping your head dropped and your arms straight.
- Breathe in and hold the position.

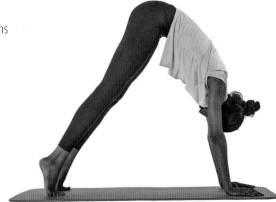

- Breathe out as you push your heels back down into the floor.
- Breathe in and hold that stretch.
- Breathe out and repeat the foot movements for 4 repetitions in total.
- Come back down on to your hands and knees and into the Extended Child's Pose (opposite).

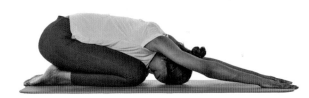

Note
- Keep your weight evenly distributed between your feet and arms.
- Try not to tense your shoulders.

Modify
- Bend your knees if you find the stretch in the legs too intense.

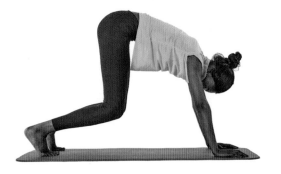

EXTENDED CHILD'S POSE

Running benefits

This is another yoga-based stretch suitable for aching shoulders and lower back which can be performed post-run or as a relief stretch between exercises. It's also a wonderful position to rest and relax in as it lengthens the spine and releases any post-run tension.

Method

- Come on to all fours with your knees under your hips and hands aligned under your shoulders.
- Sit back and let your buttocks rest on your heels.
- Lengthen your arms out in front of you, palms pressing down, and let your head rest on the floor.

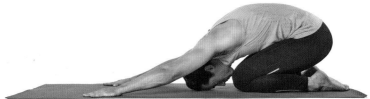

- Hold the position.
- Breathe in through your nose and in to your rib cage and then slowly out through your mouth. Stay focused as you repeat for 5 breaths, relaxing into the position.
- Stretch your arms as far forwards as you can to lengthen the muscles and stretch the upper back.

Note

- You might find that your back won't let go if it's very tight as it will be protecting itself – so take time with this exercise and don't force anything. If in any doubt, modify.
- If you have serious knee problems, avoid this exercise and instead lie on your side curled forwards.

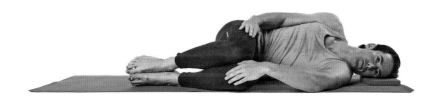

▶

Modify

- A tight lower back can prevent you from comfortably sitting back on your heels: try placing a cushion on your calves and gently sink your bottom down onto it.

- Stiff knees can also make this position uncomfortable: try placing a rolled-up towel in the crook of your knee to relieve the tension as you sit gently back.

- If you find it challenging to get into the full position, move your knees apart a little but keep your toes touching. This will enable you to sink down lower and in between your legs to rest on the floor – in this position your adductors (inner thighs) will also get a stretch.

> Pilates has benefited my running, training and overall fitness. Sometimes I run 50+ miles a week and sometimes less but my overall fitness very rarely changes. I have been doing regular Pilates for about a year and I have been injury-free. When I miss Pilates, my running suffers.
>
> Paul Buckle, ultra marathon runner

COBRA STRETCH

Running benefits

A yoga-inspired exercise to stretch and open out the chest, abdominal muscles and the hips. While running and during a Pilates session we are working our abdominal muscles hard. They need to stretch but it's not a part of the anatomy that runners often think of stretching, generally concentrating time on the legs. This exercise also strengthens and mobilizes the spine, easing out sore and tight backs — another stretch to add to your post-run repertoire.

Method

- Lie on your front.
- Take your arms out to the side and bend your elbows up to the same height as your shoulders.
- Place the palms down.

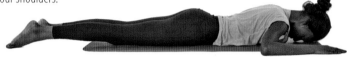

- Engage your abdominal/pelvic floor muscles.
- Breathe in to prepare.
- Breathe out and gently lift your spine slowly off the floor and extend the elbows, placing your weight on your hands.
- Lift as far as you comfortably can, lengthening your neck and fixing your gaze ahead.

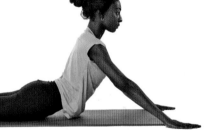

- Breathe in as you hold the stretch. Breathe out and slowly lower yourself back down to the floor. Repeat 6 times, holding for longer at the top if it feels comfortable to do so.

Note

- Keep your abdominal muscles engaged and your hips on the floor.
- Relax your shoulders and lengthen your neck, keeping it aligned.
- Concentrate on your breathing to help the movements flow.

Modify

Bend your elbows if you feel the stretch is too strong for your back.

SIDE SERIES

If you find it uncomfortable to lie on your side because your hips dig into the floor or mat, place a small towel under the area to make yourself more comfortable.

SIDE KICKS

Running benefits

All four of the following Side Kick exercises work on your core muscles, specifically your oblique (waist) muscles and hip area. These smaller waist muscles can tire more easily than the big abdominal muscles when we run. By strengthening them, there will be less side-to-side twisting of the torso, which can occur particularly when the body is flagging towards the end of a long run. The stronger the oblique muscles, the less likelihood of pelvis and hip problems. You'll also find that these exercises strengthen and lengthen the tensor fasciae latae (TFL) and iliotibial band (ITB). The TFL sits at the top of the ITB to the front, by the side of your hip – it's the muscle that stabilizes the knee and flexes, abducts and rotates the hip joint, so we need to keep it happy!

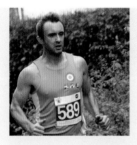

CASE STUDY

Alex Hardy runs for Ravens and Hampstead Triathlon Club. He ran his first marathon in 2015 in 3hr 14mins.

After playing football and going to the gym for most of my life, about three and a half years ago I stopped playing and started competing in triathlons. The demands on my body due to the change in training made me feel tight, I also suffered from a few minor injuries. I'd suffered from hamstring issues playing football and had been encouraged to have regular sports massages and to consider Pilates. But it was the move to triathlons with my primary focus being on running that really highlighted the need for core strength and conditioning but without the need for additional muscle mass. I also think turning 30 made a difference as I decided that I wanted to exercise for life and was concerned with my posture from constantly sitting at a desk.

Once I started attending Pilates classes I noticed real improvements in my flexibility and posture. I've suffered from fewer injuries as a consequence. I've read a lot of material on running and triathlons and I am a firm advocate that Pilates plus sports massages should be in every athlete's training regime. I'd also advocate the mental benefits of Pilates as I really do believe there's more to gain than just physical improvements – focusing on relaxation being one of them.

SIDE KICK 1 (ALL LEVELS)

Method
- Lie on your side.
- Lengthen your underneath arm directly under your head and place your head on a block or small cushion which you can balance on the upper part of your arm.

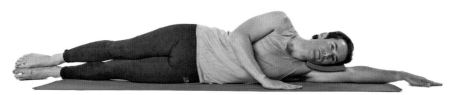

- Glance down towards your feet, check that your hips, knees and ankles are stacked and aligned.
- Place your other hand in front of your torso on the floor for support.
- Engage your abdominal/pelvic floor muscles.
- Breathe in to prepare.
- As you breathe out, raise both legs together in a straight line off the floor.

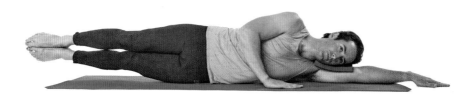

- Breathe in and hold the raised position.
- As you breathe out, slowly lower the legs, with control, down to the floor.
- Repeat 10 times.
- Turn over and perform the exercise on the other side.

Note
- The reason the block or small cushion is placed under your ear on your upper arm is to keep your neck and spine aligned.
- Try not to push your supporting hand down into the floor; keep the arm and shoulder relaxed.
- Concentrate on your breathing to keep the movements flowing and to avoid any jerky actions.

Progress
- Use ankle weights on one or both legs, but make sure you keep the lengthened alignment during the exercise.
- Increase repetitions as you become more comfortable with the exercise.

SIDE KICK 2 + INNER THIGH (ALL LEVELS)

For running benefits, see Side Kick 1 (page 88).

Method

- Lie on your side.
- Lengthen your underneath arm directly under your head and place your head on a block or small cushion which you can balance on the upper part of your arm.

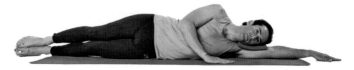

- Glance down towards your feet, check that your hips, knees and ankles are stacked and aligned.
- Place your other hand in front of your torso on the floor for support.
- Engage your abdominal/pelvic floor muscles.
- Breathe in to prepare.
- As you breathe out, raise both legs together in a straight line off the floor.

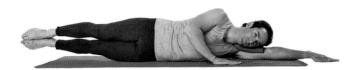

- Breathe in and hold the raised position.
- Breathe out and lift the top leg higher.

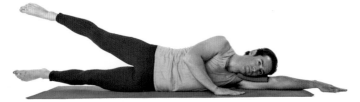

- Breathe in and hold the position.
- Breathe out and lower the top leg down to join the lower leg.
- Return both legs to floor.
- Repeat 10 times and continue with the following Inner Thigh exercise before turning over and performing the exercise on the other side.

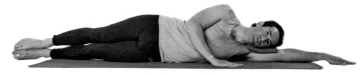

Inner thigh

- Breathe in to prepare.
- Breathe out and raise both legs together in a straight line off the floor.
- Point your toes.
- Breathe in and hold the position.

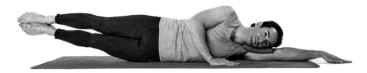

- Breathe out and raise your top leg slightly higher.
- Breathe in and hold the position.
- Breathe out and lift your lower leg up to meet the leg above.
- Breathing naturally, continue to lift and lower the underneath leg for 10 repetitions.

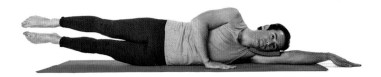

Note

- If you find the breathing challenging, just concentrate on engaging your abdominals and balancing to begin with. Breathe naturally until you get into a rhythm.
- Try not to press the supporting hand down in front of your torso – keep the rest of the body relaxed.
- Be aware of what your shoulders are doing. Keep them stabilized.

Modify

Perform fewer repetitions.

Progress

Perform more repetitions.

Use ankle weights on both ankles or just the lower leg that's working the inner thigh.

Take your supporting hand on to your upper thigh, challenging your balance further.

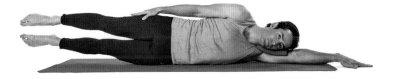

SIDE KICK 3 INTO THE TORPEDO (INTERMEDIATE)

Running benefits
As for the previous two Side Kicks (pages 88 and 90), but the Torpedo encourages and improves torso stability even more because of the arm extension.

Method
- Lie on your side.
- Lengthen your underneath arm directly under your head and place your head on a block or small cushion which you can balance on the upper part of your arm.

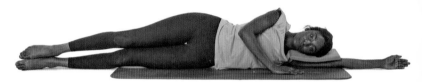

- Glance down towards your feet, check that your hips, knees and ankles are stacked and aligned.
- Engage your abdominal/pelvic floor muscles.
- Take your supporting hand and rest it, lengthening your arm as you do so, along your top thigh.

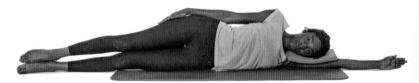

- Breathe in to prepare.
- Breathe out as you simultaneously raise both legs and extend your top arm over your head into the Torpedo position.

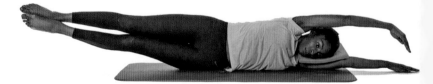

- Point your toes.
- Hold the position as you breathe in.
- Breathe out as you return your legs and arm to the starting position.
- Repeat 10 times on each side.

Note

• Focus on lengthening your legs and arms as you perform the exercise and keeping your abdominal muscles engaged.

• Use your breathing to help the exercise flow and try to avoid any jerky body movements.

Progress

• Hold a small hand weight as you extend your arm over your head and/or use ankle weights on your legs. But make sure you can still perform the exercise well, keeping the torso aligned and stable.

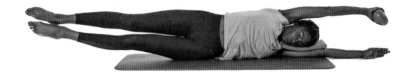

Pilates cured my chronic back pain and allowed me to start running at the age of 45. I love how if I start to feel like I am struggling with heavy legs and/or breathing when running, I can switch on my core and it's the most amazing feeling, my legs just start working in a natural and comfortable way, and I feel lighter and stronger instantly.

Sally Harvey, recreational runner

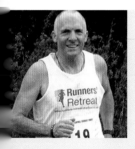

CASE STUDY

Brian Bower is a Boston Marathon qualifier, GFA London Marathon runner, and previously a GB Duathlete and Ironman.

I've run for most of my life. Now, as a mature runner I was really surprised by the immediate benefits gained when I started attending a Pilates class a little while ago. My movement and stride length improved and the relaxation aspect was phenomenal. My shoulders immediately felt less tense and the stretching means that after a Pilates class I always sleep better than normal.

SIDE KICK 4 + HAMSTRING STRETCH (INTERMEDIATE/ADVANCED)

Running benefits

In addition to the benefits listed for the previous Side Kicks (pages 88 to 92), this exercise provides an extra and quite strong hamstring stretch as well as strengthening the core, hip flexors and ankles. It also strengthens and lengthens the ITB and abductors (outside of thigh); the ITB is a very important tendon as it stabilizes the leg during running and helps extend the knee, moving the hip sideways.

Method

- Lie on your side.
- Lengthen your underneath arm directly under your head and place your head on a block or small cushion which you can balance on the upper part of your arm.
- Place your supporting hand in front of you on the floor and keep your arm relaxed.

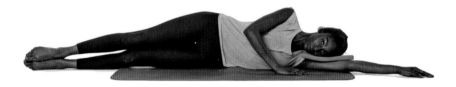

- Engage your abdominal/pelvic floor muscles.
- Breathe in to prepare and raise your upper leg so that it is just level with the top of your pelvis.
- Flex your top foot.

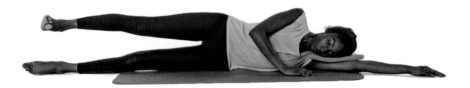

- Breathe out and sweep your leg forwards until you feel a stretch in your hamstrings.
- Pulse for two beats.

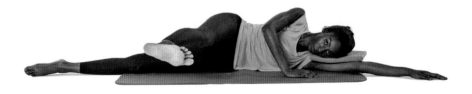

- Breathe in and sweep the leg backwards just beyond your hip joint while pointing your toe.
- Repeat 10 times and then turn over to change legs.

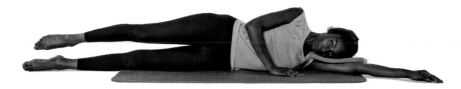

Note

- When you're performing the sweeping movement try to keep your hips and pelvis stable; they will want to follow the leg. This is challenging, so take it slowly and use your breathing to help the exercise flow.
- Keep your abdominal muscles engaged throughout.
- Be aware of any tension in your shoulders, supporting arm and hand – try to keep them relaxed.

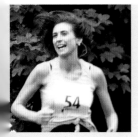

CASE STUDY

Helen Kennedy, 40, is a busy GP and recreational runner.

I have only been running for about three years, having done hardly any exercise ever before and certainly had never enjoyed exercising. I have now run three half-marathons. I took up Pilates about a year after I started to run regularly and whilst I usually only get the chance to do one session per week and would like to do more, I have noticed a big improvement in my running. Gently stretching out all my muscles feels so good and often little aches and pains from running feel so much better after Pilates. I feel stronger, taller, more upright and less slouchy when I'm running and even just walking around. I'm generally more conscious of my posture, my pelvic floor and my core too. Even the control of breathing that you learn with Pilates is helpful and I'm sure it has increased my tidal volume and ability to oxygenate my working muscles. Running with a better posture has led to me having far less problems with my lower back, which used to ache terribly if I ran more than a few miles. I also used to get a lot of pain around the insertion of my ITB on the lateral side of both my knees and since doing more Pilates, this has not been a problem. I feel that having good core strength makes me less likely to get injured, especially on uneven, off-road terrain as I can adapt and correct myself more easily so I run with more confidence and more enjoyment. My favourite exercises are the abdominal ones as this has always been the one part of my body, through vanity of wanting a flat stomach, that I have ever bothered to exercise! I love the fact that so many of the exercises have different levels so you can really challenge yourself, however strong, or not, you are feeling that day. While leg strengthening is obviously important for running, doing the variety of exercises in Pilates that include the upper body is also important to keep some balance and not neglect my arms and chest which would not really be challenged by running alone. I think that for me, the combination of regular running and Pilates achieves everything that I want in terms of keeping cardiovascularly fit, strong, toned and happy.

SIDE BEND (SIDE PLANK) (ADVANCED)

Running benefits

The Side Bend not only challenges your core stability but will also, over time, improve your running strength and stamina. As with the previous Side Kick exercises you'll find your oblique muscles working hard; this exercise will strengthen the muscles and so prevent unnecessary twisting when running. The Side Bend also works the shoulders, the supporting arm and improves hip mobility.

Note: the Side Bend can be challenging so please modify if necessary and adapt accordingly.

Method

- Sit on your right buttock, leaning on your right arm.
- Place your hand flat on the floor, slightly wider than your shoulder.

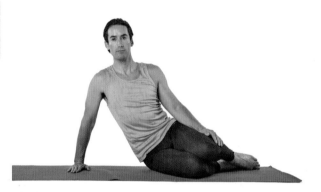

- Bend both knees to your side, heels in line with your torso.
- Bring your left foot to the front of your right foot.

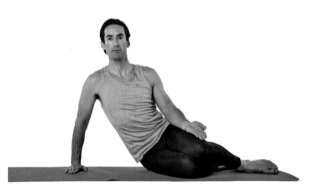

- Take your left arm and rest it on your left thigh, palm up.
- Engage your abdominal/pelvic floor muscles.
- Keep your chest open and lengthen through your spine.
- Breathe in to prepare.
- Breathe out and extend your legs away from you in a straight line as you raise up your pelvis and reach your top arm over your head into the Side Bend position.
- Breathe in again as you balance and hold the pose.

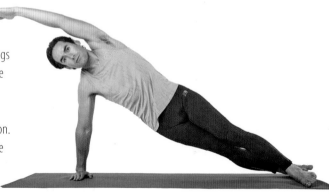

- Breathe out, bend both knees as you lower yourself slowly, with control, back to the floor, bringing your top arm down to rest at the same time.
- Repeat 4 times each side.

Note

- Try not to let your hips sag or drop down: keep them lifted, stable and facing forwards.
- Keep your abdominal muscles engaged throughout.
- Concentrate on your breathing and lengthening through your legs and arm as you perform the exercise.

Modify

- Lean on your elbow instead of lengthened arm.
- Keep your knees bent to your side throughout the exercise.
- Lift your pelvis off the floor from the bent knee position without extending your legs and stretch your arm over your head.

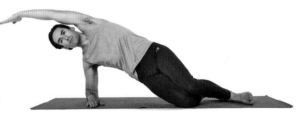

Progress

Come into the full Side Bend position with lengthened legs. Extend your arm above your body instead of over your head.

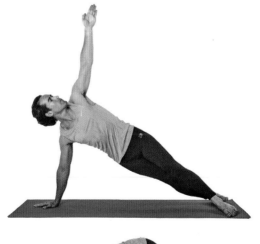

Breathe in to prepare. Breathe out and curl your arm down and under your torso, rotating your spine as you do so, 'threading the needle'.

Repeat the 'threading the needle' movement 4 times before lowering yourself, bending your knees, slowly down to the floor. Increase repetitions for further progressions.

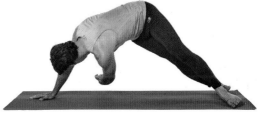

CLAM/LATERAL HIP OPENER (ALL LEVELS)

Running benefits
This exercise is a must for all runners. It targets your gluteus medius muscle, the middle-sized buttock muscle that works to encourage pelvic and knee stability. If this muscle becomes tight or shortened then the pelvic instability it causes can lead to lower back ache, knee and hip problems. It's an excellent exercise for the ITB and TFL as well because it lengthens them both along with the hip rotators (which includes the piriformis, which can sometimes cause problems for runners – see page 186). In addition, the Clam can often help with sciatic pain and hamstring strain.

Method
- Lie on your side.
- Lengthen your underneath arm directly under your head and place your head on a block or small cushion which you can balance on the upper part of your arm.
- Bend both knees and keep your heels in line with your buttocks.
- Engage your abdominal/pelvic floor muscles.

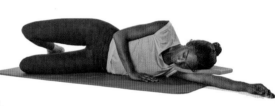

- Breathe naturally.
- Raise your top knee just a small amount, keeping your feet on the floor.
- Return your knee to the starting position.
- Repeat up to 16 times and then change sides.

Note
- Keep your feet glued together throughout and your torso stable.
- If you feel your pelvis rotating backwards then you are opening up your knee too far. Keep the movement small.

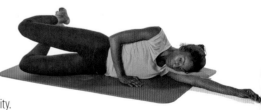

Progress
- Lift the feet off the floor behind you, keeping your heels in line with your bottom.
- Repeat the same knee-opening movement in this position, making sure you maintain the pelvic stability. It's just a small movement to activate the gluteus medius muscle; don't let the pelvis rotate backwards.
- Repeat 10 times.
- On the last repetition hold the knee open and gentl pulse the knee upwards 10 times.
- Change sides and repeat.

OUTER AND INNER THIGH LIFTS (ALL LEVELS)

OUTER THIGH LIFTS (ABDUCTOR MUSCLES)

Running benefits

This is not a classic Pilates exercise but one well worth including in a book on Pilates for runners. This exercise will not only strengthen the outer thigh, ITB and glutes but also improve your running form and posture. Strong quads and glutes will help you to fly up those hills! Knee problems can sometimes stem from quadricep imbalances which could cause patella (knee cap) tracking issues. The quadriceps are the muscles at the front of the thigh which help keep the knee cap stable - so this is another good reason to strengthen those thigh muscles. This exercise, like all the side-lying exercises, also challenges balance and strengthens the core muscles.

Method

- Lie on your side.
  Lengthen your underneath arm directly under your head and place your head on a block or small cushion which you can balance on the upper part of your arm.
  Place your other hand in front of you on the floor for support.
  Check that you are in neutral spine and make sure your body is in a straight line, hips, knees and ankles stacked.
  Bend your underneath leg in front of you.
  Lengthen your top leg, rotating your foot so that your toes face slightly downwards.

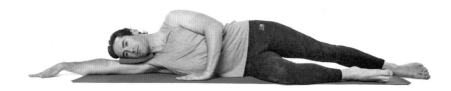

Engage your abdominal/pelvic floor muscles.
Breathe in to your rib cage to prepare.
Breathe out and raise your top leg, keeping it lengthened and long.

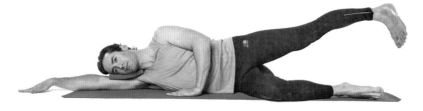

Breathe out and lower the leg but let it hover above the underneath leg, don't relax it.

▶

- Repeat 16 times in total and then follow it with the Inner Thigh Lift (page 101).

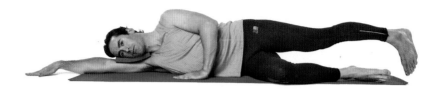

Note

- Be aware of your pelvic stability – make sure there is no wobble. If there is, don't take your leg so high.
- Relax your shoulders and your supporting arm; try not to take any tension in the upper body.
- Concentrate on your breathing to help the exercise flow and avoid jerky movements.
- Keep your abdominal muscles engaged throughout.

Progress (advanced)

- Increase repetitions.
- Take your supporting arm and lengthen it along your top thigh as you lift. This will challenge your balance.
- Use ankle weights as long as you can keep your body aligned.

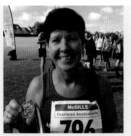

CASE STUDY

Andrea Holmes from Worcestershire has been running for two and a half years: parkruns, 5ks, 10ks and a half marathon. She runs mainly for health, fitness and enjoyment.

As my 50th birthday loomed, I decided to set myself some challenges, one of which was to start running. I now run approximately three times a week, mainly as part of a running group session but sometimes on my own – running gives me time to switch off and feel free. I started Pilates to strengthen my core and to feel stretched and looser … I've had back problems in the past but not since I started Pilates. I found it made a real difference to my running – when I start to feel like my body is 'sagging' I envisage a host of helium balloons lifting my head up and that does the trick perfectly. I feel my posture is upright and strong again! Core strength then allows me to feel stable and secure when running, balance is much improved too. I can now run for longer and feel stronger, this in turn, I'm sure, has made a difference to my stamina and tackling those hills! Running leaves me invigorated, buzzing, feeling like I have had a good workout, while Pilates leaves me relaxed, stretched, looser.

INNER THIGH LIFTS

Running benefits

This exercise accompanies the Outer Thigh Lifts (page 99) and it's important to practise them together. The benefits are the same, although this exercise will strengthen the adductor muscles (inner thigh) and increase pelvic stability.

Method

- Lie on your side.
- Lengthen your underneath arm directly under your head and place your head on a block or small cushion which you can balance on the upper part of your arm.
- Place your other hand in front of you on the floor for support.
- Check that you are in neutral spine and make sure your body is in a straight line, hips, knees and ankles stacked.
- Bend your top leg and take the knee on to the floor in front of you.
- Lengthen your underneath leg and point your toes.

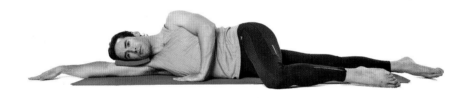

Engage your abdominal/pelvic floor muscles.

Breathe in to prepare.

Breathe out and raise your lower leg, lengthening it away, pointing your toes.

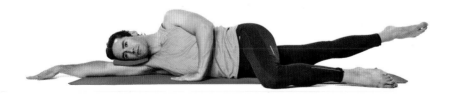

Breathe in and lower the leg but let it hover above the floor; don't let the muscles relax.

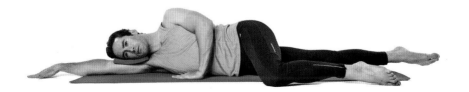

▶

- Breathe out and lift again.
- Repeat 16 times in total and then turn over and perform both this exercise and the Outer Thigh Lift (page 99) on the other side.

Note

- Be aware of pelvic stability – if you find that your pelvis rolls forwards because your top leg is pulling it towards the floor, place a cushion underneath your front knee to raise it up.
- Relax your shoulders and your supporting arm; try not to take any tension in the upper body.
- Keep your abdominal muscles engaged throughout.

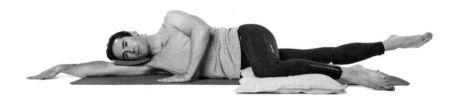

Progress (advanced)

- Increase repetitions.
- Use ankle weights as long as you can keep your body aligned.

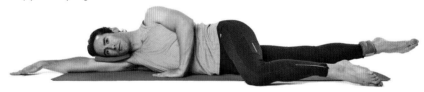

> Pilates has definitely had a positive effect on my running. Over the years I developed quite a bad posture and running long distances inevitably resulted in many aches and pains. Regular Pilates has really helped me to improve my posture generally, and has noticeably reduced my neck and shoulder pain when running those longer distances, making me a much stronger and efficient runner.
>
> Victoria Field, marathon runner

CHEST OPENER

Running benefits

This exercise can be performed either as a post-run stretch or during your regular Pilates session. It opens out the chest, stretching the pectoral muscles, which can become tight as your shoulders hunch forwards when tired during a run. Having an open chest when running means your lungs can work more efficiently. As you rotate in this exercise you'll be improving the mobility of your thoracic spine (page 27), strengthening the back muscles. Your shoulders will also get a good stretch, increasing flexibility and so improving arm drive.

Method

- Lie on your side with knees bent and your heels in line with your buttocks.
- Place a block or small cushion under your ear to keep your neck and spine aligned.
- Lengthen your underneath arm along the floor in front of your chest, palm up.
- Bring your other arm to rest on top of the lower arm, palms together.

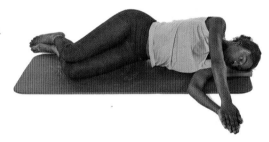

- Engage your abdominal/pelvic floor muscles.

- Breathe in to prepare.
- Breathe out and raise your top arm up towards the ceiling at the same time as rotating your spine.

Take the arm as far back as you can, your head, neck and spine following it.
Breathe in as you hold the open rotation.
Breathe out and return slowly to the start position.
Repeat 6 times and then roll over to perform the exercise on the other side.

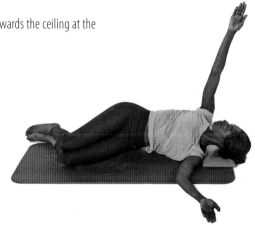

Note

- Keep your hips stacked; don't let your pelvis rotate back with your spine, it needs to stay put.

Modify

- If the rotation is challenging and your chest muscles are very tight, just take your arm above and in line with your chest instead of rotating behind. Over time, as you work on your spinal flexibility you will find that you'll be able to rotate further.

FRONT SERIES

SINGLE KNEE FOLD (BEGINNER/INTERMEDIATE)

Running benefits

This exercise teaches a very basic pelvic and torso stability. It is also a good hip mobility exercise and strengthens the lumbar spine (page 27). Although this feels like a simple exercise, it is a good one to start with and relates well to running – you are lifting alternate legs while keeping the torso stable and so mimicking the running motion. While performing the exercise, pay special attention to what your pelvis is doing – does it lift up or shift? Keep those abdominal muscles engaged and you will notice a difference.

Method

- Lie on your back.
- Place a block or small cushion under your head to keep your neck and spine aligned.
- Take your arms down by your sides and keep them relaxed.
- Bend your knees.

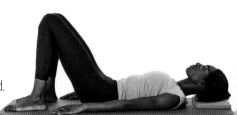

- Make sure you're in neutral spine – perform a few pelvic tilts to find the correct position and then relax.
- Place your feet in line with your hips.
- Engage your abdominal/pelvic floor muscles.
- Breathe in to your rib cage to prepare.
- Breathe out through your mouth while raising your right leg into the tabletop position.
- Your knee is directly over your hip and your shin is parallel to the ceiling.
- Point your toes.

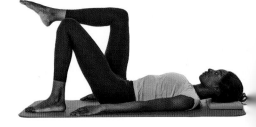

- Breathe in and, keeping your leg in this 90-degree angle and moving from the hip, lower your foot slowly and smoothly to the ground.

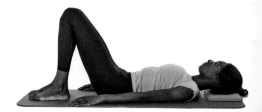

- Breathe out and return the leg, with control, to the tabletop position.
- Repeat for a total of 4 times either side.

Note

- Pay attention to your pelvis: make sure it's not moving around and that your back isn't arching as you lower your leg to the floor.
- Keep your abdominal muscles engaged and the rest of your body relaxed with your shoulders down in your back pockets.
- Concentrate on your breathing to help the exercise flow.

DOUBLE KNEE FOLD (INTERMEDIATE/ADVANCED)

This is a progression from the Single Knee Fold. Make sure you can perform the Single Knee Fold and are comfortable with the process before moving on to this exercise.

Method

- Lie on your back.
- Place a block or small cushion under your head to keep your neck and spine aligned.
- Take your arms down by your sides and keep them relaxed.
- Bend your knees.
- Place your feet in line with your hips.
- Perform a few pelvic tilts and come into neutral spine or imprint (page 28).
- Engage your abdominal muscles/pelvic floor muscles.
- Breathe in to your rib cage to prepare.
- Breathe out and raise your right leg into the tabletop position.

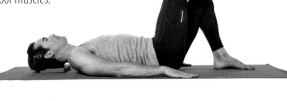

- Breathe in and hold.
- Breathe out and raise your left leg into the tabletop position.

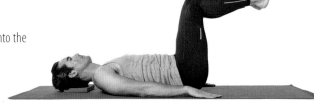

- Make sure both your knees are sitting above your hips.
- Point your toes.
- Breathe in to prepare.
- Breathe out and lower your right foot to the floor, keeping the 90-degree angle of the leg.

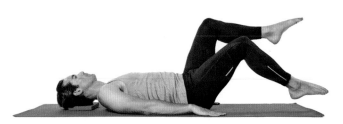

Breathe in and return it to the start position.
Breathe out and lower your left foot to the floor.
Breathe in and return it to the start position.
Continue alternating for a total of up to 8 repetitions.
When you've completed the exercise, take one foot down to the mat at a time so that you don't arch your back.

▶

Note

- Check that your abdominal muscles aren't doming as you perform the exercise and that your back isn't arching. Keep your abdominal muscles activated throughout.

- If you find your back beginning to arch, don't take your foot down so low — stop halfway until you feel stronger. Don't allow the knee joint to move.

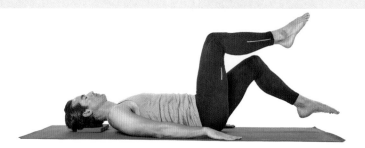

> I had many injuries and was constantly in pain from something after starting on marathons three years ago. To complicate matters I am hypermobile. I started 'synergy' (Pilates/yoga fusion) a year ago and have managed 62 marathons/ultras since January 2015 with no real injury issues. Coincidence, maybe, but I'll keep going!
>
> Carolyn Thomson Easter, ultra marathon runner

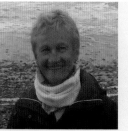

CASE STUDY

Marina Knibbe has been running regularly for 14 years, both for fitness and because she says she is addicted! She has so far run 10k and 10-mile races and is aiming to run some half marathons. She practises Pilates three to four times a week and her favourite runs are 10k trail runs.

Pilates has helped my running enormously by making me more aware of the different muscle groups in my body and how I can strengthen them to make me a better runner, to give me more stamina and to keep injuries at bay and the importance of good glutes! I would recommend Pilates as a way in to exercise for anyone who is wanting to improve their fitness, but has not done any exercise before, as well as for people who want to improve their core strength. It has a 'feel good' factor too which should not be underestimated.

ANKLE MOBILITY (ALL LEVELS)

Running benefits

A simple but important exercise to achieve and maintain full range of movement and improve strength in the ankles and feet. Your feet and ankles have to withstand the impact of running, and this exercise, and those that follow, will help them to do so. You can also perform this exercise standing up if you prefer, as part of the balance routine. The pointing and flexing of the foot improves flexibility and also stretches and lengthens the muscles of the front and then the back of the leg. If you're short of time, instead of lying on your back, perform the exercises while you're sitting at your desk or whenever you are sat down!

Method

- Lie on your back.
- Place a block or small cushion under your head to keep your neck and spine aligned.
- Take your arms down by your sides and keep them relaxed.
- Bend your knees.
- Place your feet in line with your hips.
- Perform a few pelvic tilts and come into neutral spine.
- Engage your abdominal/pelvic floor muscles.
- Breathe naturally and raise your right leg up into the tabletop position.

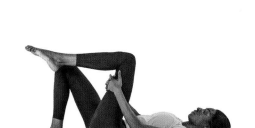

- Place your hands lightly around your raised thigh to support the leg.
- Rotate your ankle very slowly in one direction 6 times, and then reverse it.
- Return your foot to centre, then alternate pointing your toes and flexing your foot 6 times.

- Change legs and repeat the exercise using the other leg.

Note

- Try to draw a full circle with your toes when rotating from your ankle.
- Keep the knee and lower leg stable. Don't let it circle with your foot.
- Relax your shoulders. Be aware of the rest of your body – is it trying to join in?

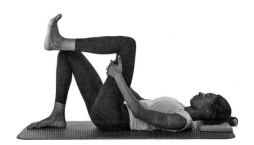

SHOULDER STABILITY (ALL LEVELS)

Running benefits

The following simple and relaxing exercises will train your shoulders to stay in a neutral position. This will transfer to your running by reducing the tension that can sometimes be felt in the shoulder area. You will also be stretching your trapezius muscles (upper back) and mobilizing your shoulder blades, ensuring your shoulders move more freely on a run. If you perform these exercises with light hand weights (see progressions) then you will also be strengthening your arms, which in turn will improve your running drive.

Method

- Lie on your back.
- Bend your knees, feet in line with your hips.
- Come into neutral spine.
- Breathe naturally.
- Raise your arms straight up above your chest with palms facing.

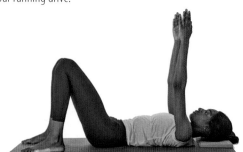

- Engage your abdominal/pelvic floor muscles.
- Gently lift your shoulders off the floor as if you're trying to reach the ceiling with your fingertips.

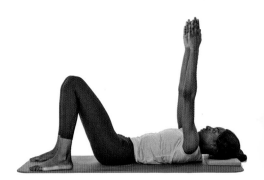

- Keeping your arms fully lengthened, shrug your shoulders gently back down to the floor.
- Repeat the movement slowly, 10 times in total.
- Return to the start position ready to go into the Arms and Shoulders exercise opposite.

Note

- Be aware of the rest of your body – when you lift your arms and shoulders, make sure the rest of the torso isn't going with you and that it stays stable.
- Try not to crash your shoulders back down on to the floor; keep the exercise flowing and controlled.
- Keep your neck and head stable.

Progress

- Use light hand weights.

ARMS AND SHOULDERS

Note: if you have shoulder problems, please modify.

Method

- Lie on your back.
- Bend your knees, feet in line with your hips.
- Come into neutral spine.
- Breathe naturally.
- Raise your arms straight up above your chest with palms facing.

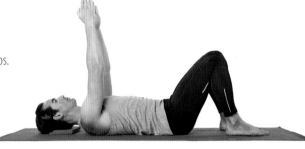

- Engage your abdominal/pelvic floor muscles.
- Breathe in to prepare.
- Breathe out and lengthen your right arm back behind your head, taking it level with your ear (no further) and simultaneously take your left arm down by your side.

- Breathe in and hold the position.
- Breathe out and, keeping the movement smooth, swap the arms over.
- Repeat for a total of 10 times. Return to the start position ready to go into Arms, Shoulders and Spinal Mobility (page 110).

Note

- Keep your torso stable, remain in neutral spine and make sure you do not arch your back as you take an arm back.
- Try and straighten your arms, stretching the triceps (back of the arms) in the process, but keep your elbow slightly soft.
- Make sure your arm doesn't hug your head as you take it back – leave a space between your shoulder and your ear. Think about the alignment.

Modify

If you have shoulder problems and it's not comfortable to take your arm back level with your ear, just take it to a comfortable position – don't force it.

Progress

- Use light hand weights

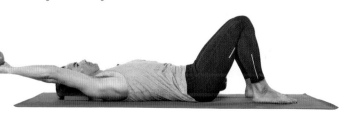

ARMS, SHOULDERS AND SPINAL MOBILITY

Method

- Lie on your back.
- Bend your knees, feet in line with your hips.
- Come into neutral spine.
- Breathe naturally.
- Raise your arms straight up above your chest with palms facing.
- Engage your abdominal/pelvic floor muscles.
- Breathe in to prepare.
- Breathe out and take both arms back behind your head no further than your ears.

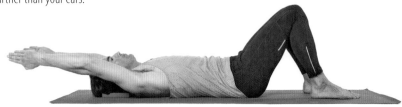

- Breathe in and hold the stretch but keep your torso in neutral spine.
- Breathe out and bring your arms back above your chest and then lower both down to your sides.
- Repeat for a total of 10 times.
- Return your arms to the centre ready to go into Arm Circles (opposite).

Note

- Be aware of any spinal arching – your back will want to arch as you take both arms back.
- Keep your abdominals engaged and your spine stable.
- If you find your back is beginning to arch and your ribs lift up then don't take your arms so far back.

Progress

- Use light hand weights but pay special attention to your alignment. Your back will want to arch against the weight of your hands even more now, so keep your spine in neutral and down on the floor and your abdominal muscles engaged.

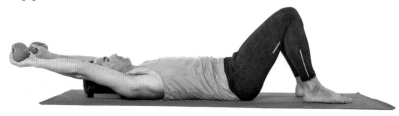

RM CIRCLES

ınning benefits

ım circles improve both shoulder mobility and stabilization. This exercise will also challenge the steadiness of ur torso, as it may want to move with your arms – it is a great exercise for training it to stay stable while we ɔve our arms, which is what we want it to do when we run. You'll also find your arm swing will improve as the ɔulders become more flexible and mobile.

ote: if you have a shoulder problem, please keep ıese rotations small or omit the exercise.

ethod

Lie on your back in neutral spine.
Bend your knees, feet in line with your hips.
Breathe naturally.
Raise your arms straight up above your chest with palms facing.

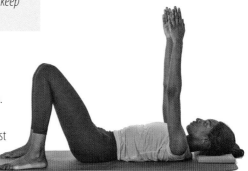

Engage your abdominal/pelvic floor muscles.
Begin rotating both arms from the shoulders, drawing a circle on the ceiling with your fingertips.
Rotate in one direction a few times, then rotate the other way.
Come back to centre and stop circling.

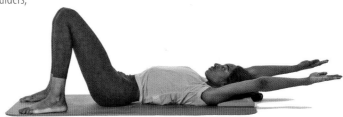

Breathe in to your rib cage.
Breathe out through your mouth as you begin to make the circles bigger.
Keep the lateral thoracic breathing going as you increase the range of movement, taking the arms behind your head and all the way round to your sides and then back up above your chest.

Make a full circle on each breath.
Complete 5 circles and then change direction.

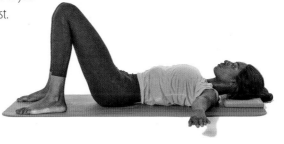

▶

Note

- Keep your abdominals engaged and your spine stable.
- If you find your back is beginning to arch and your ribs lift up then keep the rotations small.
- Keep the rest of the body relaxed and centred as you perform the Arm Circles.

I love the Roll Down because it is so relaxing and at the same time gives such a good stretch. But I also love all the exercises which target the abs, especially with the weighted balls.

Marina Knibbe, self-confessed running addict

Progress

- Use light hand weights, but make sure you stay in neutral spine and that the weights don't alter your exercise form or alignment.
- Increase the repetitions and range of movement but don't take the arms further back than your ears.

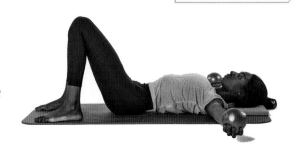

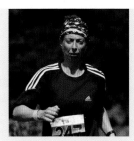

CASE STUDY

Jane Holt from Staffordshire, who runs for Newcastle (Staffs) AC, recently completed the Millennium Way Ultra, a 41-mile race across Staffordshire. She has run six ultras and six marathons.

I have had recurring knee injuries over the last three years and my physio recommended strength and conditioning work along with Pilates to improve my mobility. I also have the all-too-common problem of tight hip flexors/weak glutes along with poor posture, caused by too much sitting! I am a self-employed copywriter and work from home so spend far too long sat in front of a computer. This along with biomechanical faults and poor running form contributed to recurring bouts of patellofemoral pain syndrome (runner's knee) and patella tendinopathy. I started doing Pilates two years ago and it made a noticeable difference. My core/glutes became stronger and I was much more flexible and mobile. My lower back stiffness/tightness eased and my hip flexors were pliable and supple. There was an overall improvement in my posture – no 'chin poke' or shoulder slumping. I attended a class once a week on a regular basis. This was on Monday mornings, which was ideal after doing my Sunday long run or following a race. It eased any stiffness/tightness and I generally felt refreshed afterwards. The main benefit for me is postural. Extended periods of computer work have played havoc with my posture, leaving me with a tight lower back and a forward tilted pelvis that has contributed to my knee injuries. I have muscle imbalances on my right side – hence the problem with my right knee – causing a tracking problem with my kneecap (patella maltracking) and the subsequent injuries. Another positive is improved core strength and flexibility.

DEAD BUG (ALL LEVELS)

Running benefits

A relaxing exercise that lengthens nearly all the muscles in your body and helps to make you more aware of torso stability. This will transfer to your running, encouraging torso stability while your arms and legs move. Think back to the tree trunk on page 5 – the arms and legs are branches waving around and it's vital that you keep the trunk and roots stable. This exercise also strengthens the back, arm and leg muscles and can be made more challenging by using hand and leg weights.

Method

- Lie on your back.
- Place your arms down by your sides.
- Bend your knees, feet in line with your hips.
- Come into neutral spine.
  Take your right leg into the tabletop position. Raise your left arm above your chest with the palm of your hand facing inwards.

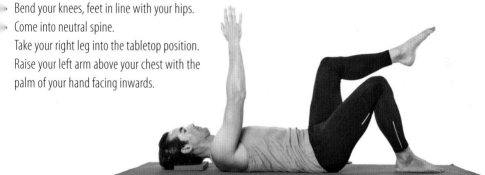

Engage your abdominal/pelvic floor muscles.
Breathe in to prepare.
Breathe out and lengthen your arm back behind your head, simultaneously extending your leg out in front of you, pointing your toes.

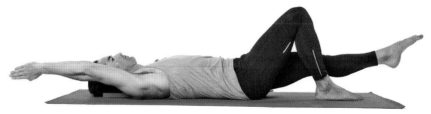

Only take your arm back level with your ear, no further.
Take your leg as low as you can but if you feel your back begin to arch, then raise your leg slightly higher.
Breathe in, holding the lengthened position.
Breathe out and slowly, with control, return the arm and leg back to the start position.

▶

- Repeat 8 times in total and then change sides.

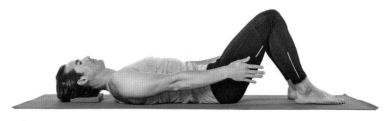

Note

- Leave a space between your ear and arm when you lengthen it – don't hug your head.
- Try to stretch your triceps (back of the arms) as you lengthen the arm but keep your elbow soft.
- Concentrate on your breathing to help the exercise flow.
- Stay in neutral spine – be aware of any change in your alignment as you move your arms and legs.

Progress

- This exercise can be performed with light arm weights, but make sure when you take your arm back that it is stable.

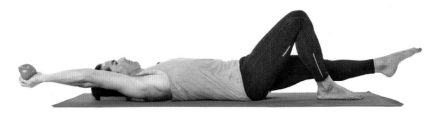

- The same applies to the legs: you can use leg weights, although I would suggest starting with just arm weights to begin with. You are more likely to feel the back arch if you are wearing a leg weight, so concentrate on keeping the pelvis stable and spine in neutral.

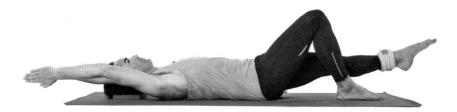

- Increase repetitions.

NECK CURL-UPS (BEGINNER)

Running benefits

These gentle Curl-Ups will introduce you to the action of activating the abdominal muscles while you raise your head, neck and shoulders. You will need to be able to do this in many of the following exercises. Neck Curl-Ups target the rectus abdominis, the potential six-pack muscles, as well as working the neck flexors.

Method

- Lie on your back.
- Bend your knees, feet in line with your hips.
- Place a block or small cushion under your head to keep your neck and spine aligned.
- Place one hand on your abdomen and take the other lightly behind your head.

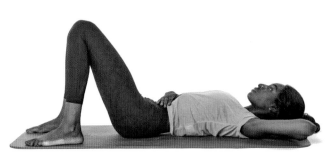

- Make sure you are in neutral spine.
- Engage your abdominal/pelvic floor muscles.
- Breathe in to prepare.
- Breathe out and gently raise your head, supported by your hand, lengthening and flexing your neck.

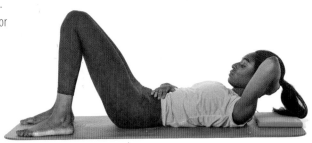

- Look towards your thighs.
- Breathe in and hold the position.
- Breathe out and lower yourself back down to the starting position.
- Repeat 6 times.

Note

- By placing your hand on your abdomen you will be able to feel the muscles activating as you curl up.
- If you feel your abdominal muscles start to bulge, return back down to the floor.
- Keep the abdominal muscles activated – pull them in before you move so that you are centred and stable and your abdominal muscles won't dome.

THE HUNDRED (PREPARATION – ALL LEVELS)

Running benefits

The Hundred is a classic mat Pilates exercise that improves circulation, deep abdominal and lumbar strength. It also enhances pelvic and shoulder stability, while challenging the leg and hip muscles. It's called The Hundred because it involves one hundred gentle beats of the arms. It's an all-over core strengthener that is a 'must' for any runner. Weak abdominals just can't support your back when running, so this is a good place to start.

Before you perform the full exercise it's a good idea to practise the preparation. The Hundred is an intense and challenging exercise and so it's important to get the process and alignment correct. Although Joseph Pilates described it as a 'warm-up exercise', I'm not sure I agree!

Method

Part 1 (all levels)

- Lie on your back, knees bent and feet in line with the hips.
- Perform a few pelvic tilts and come into neutral spine.
- Engage your abdominal/pelvic floor muscles.
- Breathe in to your rib cage to prepare.

- Breathe out as you raise your head, curling up and lengthening through your neck to fix your gaze on your thighs/pelvis.
- Lift and lengthen your arms a little way off the floor, palms down, level with your shoulders.

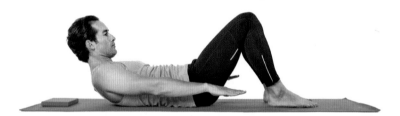

- Breathe in and hold the position.
- Breathe out and gently lower your head, neck and arms back down to the floor.
- Repeat the exercise once more and move on to part 2.

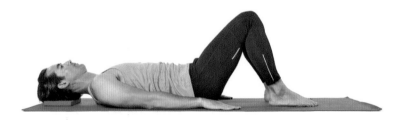

Part 2 (intermediate/advanced)

As long as you are not taking tension in your neck and you can feel your abdominal muscles working, progress to this next stage. If you have a neck problem of any sort, omit this part of the exercise.

- Lie on your back, knees bent and feet in line with the hips.
- Perform a few pelvic tilts and come into neutral spine.
- Engage your abdominal/pelvic floor muscles.
- Breathe in to prepare.

- Breathe out as you raise your head, curling up and lengthening through your neck to fix your gaze on your pelvis.
- Breathe in and raise your arms up to shoulder level, palms down.

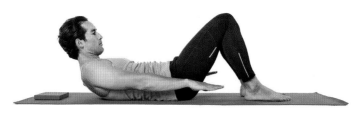

Breathe out and, keeping your head and neck in the same position, take your arms back behind you (no further than your ears) and lengthen.

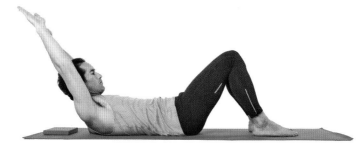

Breathe in holding the position.
Breathe out and gently lower your head, neck and arms back down to the floor and come into a full body stretch.

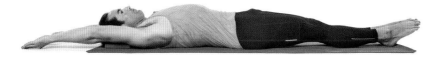

Rock your head gently from side to side to release any tension.
Repeat 2 times, as long as you are using your abdominal muscles and not straining your neck.

Note

- If you feel a lot of tension in your neck, do not take your arms back, just release down to the mat and complete the first part of this exercise.
- Engaging your abdominal muscles before you breathe in and move will help.

- Imagine you have an apple or tennis ball under your chin and you are trying to hold it there as you perform the exercise and look towards your pelvis or thighs.

THE HUNDRED (ALL LEVELS)

Method

- Lie on your back, knees bent, feet in line with the hips.
- Perform a few pelvic tilts and come into neutral spine or imprint your spine (page 28).
- Engage your abdominal/pelvic floor muscles.
- Raise one leg at a time into the tabletop position.

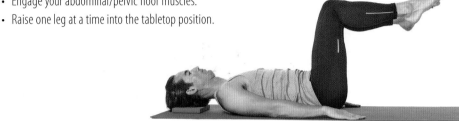

- Breathe in to prepare.
- Breathe out as you raise your head, curling up and lengthening through your neck to fix your gaze on your thighs.
- Raise your arms up to the same height as your shoulders, palms down.
- Breathe in for 5 beats as you gently pulse your arms, moving from your shoulders.

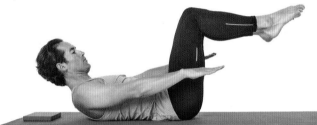

- Breathe out for 5 beats.
- Repeat until you have completed 100 gentle pulses with your arms.

Note

- If you feel tension in your neck or have a neck problem, put your head down.
- Keep those abdominal/pelvic floor muscles engaged throughout.
- Imagine you have something delicate under your hands as you pulse; keep the movement small.
- Concentrate on your breathing to help the exercise flow.

I believe a very stable core is vital for endurance runners. I teach folk just five of these exercises to do daily. It's especially important as lots of people have lower back issues.

Rory Coleman (www.rorycoleman.co.uk), trainer and life coach who has run an incredible 975 marathons, hundreds of ultras, 13 Marathon des Sables and set 9 Guinness World Records.

Modify (beginners)

- If you find 100 beats too many to start with, then aim for 50 and build up.
- Alternatively, perform the exercise without raising your head or arms. Engage the abdominal muscles and hold the legs stable in the tabletop position, making sure your back doesn't arch – you'll still be working the TVA.

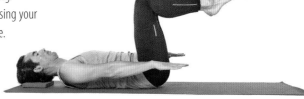

- Focus on your lateral thoracic breathing.
- When you feel strong enough, try raising your head, neck and arms for a short while.

Progress (advanced)

- With both legs in the tabletop position, raise your arms to shoulder height and your head to look towards your knees.
- Keep your abdominal muscles engaged and stay in the imprinted spine position (page 34).
- Breathe in for 5 beats of the arms and breathe out for 5 beats.
- Lengthen both legs out in front of you and lower them towards the floor. Make sure your back doesn't arch and that you keep your spine stable.

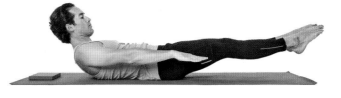

If you find your back arching, lift your legs higher.
Alternatively, lengthen one leg out in front of you at a time.

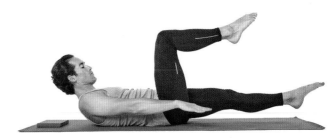

Aim for 100 beats of the arms. When you've completed the exercise, take your head and arms down to the floor followed by one leg at a time. Come into a full body stretch.

SINGLE LEG STRETCH (BEGINNER)

Running benefits

This exercise will strengthen your core muscles, increase flexibility and challenge your coordination. It stretches the hamstrings, abdominal muscles, glutes, neck and hip flexors. The hip flexors help raise the leg – think how often they have to do that on a run and how hard they need to work! If you sit at a desk all day your hip flexors (as well as your hamstrings and glutes) can become tight, so it's important to strengthen and lengthen them, as they are often neglected by runners until it's too late.

Method

- Lie on your back.
- Bend your knees, feet in line with your hips.
- Perform a few pelvic tilts to find your neutral spine.
- Engage your abdominal/pelvic floor muscles.
- Raise first your right leg and then your left leg into the tabletop position.

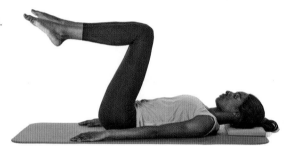

- Raise your head, lengthening through your neck so that you're looking towards your pelvis.
- Place your hands lightly either side of your right knee or calf.
- Extend your left leg out in front of you, hovering above the floor, pointing your toes.

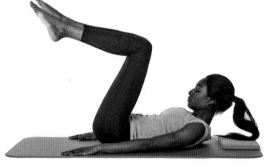

- Breathe in to prepare.
- Breathe out and swap the legs over, moving your hands from leg to leg as you do so and keeping your neck flexed as you look towards your pelvis/thighs.

- Continue slowly in a controlled manner, using lateral thoracic breathing or breathing naturally if you find it easier.

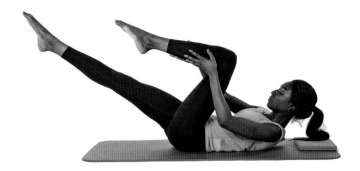

- Complete 16 repetitions. Then take your head and neck down to the floor before lowering first one leg and then the other. Come into a full body stretch.

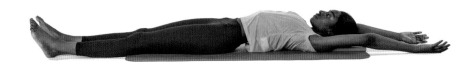

Note

- Keep your abdominal muscles engaged and be aware of any movement in your torso.
- Try and keep the rest of the body relaxed – watch your shoulders don't end up around your ears.
- Don't hold your breath – if you find the lateral thoracic breathing challenging, try short out breaths every time your leg returns.

I discovered the connection between Pilates and running a few years ago and haven't looked back since. I used to suffer from niggling injuries such as neck, hip and back pain and found this was mainly due to bad posture. When I trained for the London Marathon I made Pilates an integral part of my training plan and I am convinced that without all the stretching and strengthening exercises I would not have made it round without some sort of injury.

Sandra Davies, recreational runner

DOUBLE LEG STRETCH (INTERMEDIATE/ADVANCED)

Running benefits

This is a more challenging exercise than the Single Leg Stretch (page 120). It requires good abdominal strength and control to maintain alignment. But like the Single Leg Stretch this exercise will strengthen your core muscles, increase flexibility and challenge your coordination. It stretches the hamstrings, abdominal muscles, glutes, neck and hip flexors. When your hip flexors are lengthened, any tightness you might feel in your hamstrings, ITB or quads should start to release. In addition, this is a good shoulder mobilizer so will improve arm drive.

Note: if you have neck problems, please take care or modify.

Method

- Lie on your back, knees bent and feet in line with the hips.
- Come into neutral spine.
- Engage your abdominal/pelvic floor muscles.
- Raise first your right leg and then your left leg into the tabletop position.
- Raise your head, lengthening through your neck so that you're looking towards your knees.
- Place your hands lightly around either side of both your knees.

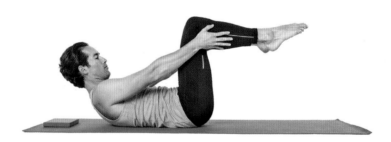

- Breathe in to your rib cage to prepare.
- Breathe out, lengthening your arms behind you as far as your ears, and simultaneously lengthening your legs out.

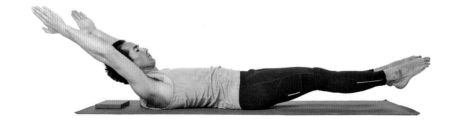

- Breathe in and return to the start position, keeping your head and neck in the flexed position.
- Breathe out and repeat the movement, lengthening your arms behind and legs out in front.
- Repeat 10 times and then bring your arms down by your sides. Lower your head, and then take one leg at a time down to the floor. Come into a full body stretch.

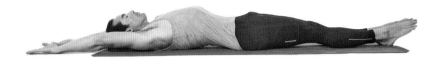

Note
- Make sure your back does not arch; keep your abdominals engaged throughout.
- If your back is arching, when lengthening lift your legs up a little higher until you are stronger.
- Keep your eyes on your knees; don't let your neck and head drop back.

Modify
- If your neck is feeling tense, take your head down to the floor.
- Take your arms only halfway back and keep your legs higher.

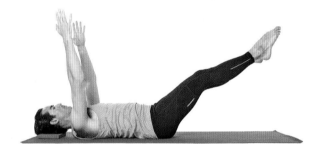

- Only extend the legs, omit the arm movement.

- Perform the Single Leg Stretch (page 120).

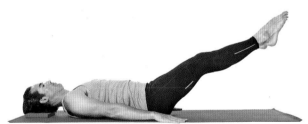

Progress
- Increase repetitions.
- Slow the exercise right down.
- Circle your arms around to the sides of your body to bring them back to the starting position, simultaneously bring your knees back to your torso.

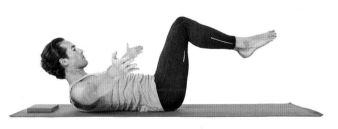

> I started attending a Pilates class really because I couldn't run at the time. What I got from my very first lesson was sleep! Yes, it was my first night of quality sleep in a while which really surprised me. Now I'm back running and I can feel the difference already from the Pilates lessons. Mainly in my posture and running form. One more thing, Pilates is not easy at all! Definitely harder than running! You engage muscles you didn't know existed. But I am a convert.
>
> Babajide Odeleye Evanson, recreational runner hoping to run a marathon soon

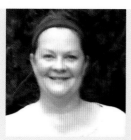

CASE STUDY

Verity West is a beginner, new to running and loving it.

Pilates has really helped me with learning how to run. As a beginner we don't always do the right thing instinctively, so have to teach our bodies. I personally have a tendency to look at the floor when I run (trying to avoid face planting), but remembering to 'run tall' definitely helps me to keep going and stop shuffling. I try to imagine I have balloons attached to the top of my head, which helps to prevent post-run back and neck pains. The core strength you build up by doing Pilates also really helps with my running posture, which, along with building strength all over the body, makes the combination of both a really useful pairing. Pilates has really helped to improve my flexibility and made me more aware of my body and what it can do. Being conscious of my posture on a daily basis has noticeably helped with the back problems I used to have. No more trips to the osteopath with back problems since doing Pilates!

SHOULDER BRIDGE (ALL LEVELS)

Running benefits

The Shoulder Bridge is another brilliant and popular exercise for runners that teaches torso stability, lengthens the spine and has the added benefit of strengthening and activating lazy glutes. As runners our glutes often let us down, either because they're not firing properly or are weak. This can cause all sorts of problems, and is often the cause of lumbar and pelvic instability (see Chapter 4). If you want to run faster, sprint those hills and have happy hamstrings – strengthen your glutes! The Shoulder Bridge also encourages spinal alignment, mobility, and stretches the back muscles and quads while strengthening the hamstrings and core muscles. It opens up the hips and lengthens the hip flexors. In other words it does everything a runner could possibly need!

It's a great exercise to do post-run as part of your cool down if you have a tight, achy back and screaming hamstrings, or even if you have been sedentary all day. It undoes all those knotty tension spots in your back. Stick to the basic beginners exercise rather than the progressions if you're just using it as a post-run stretch.

In addition, if you have a groin or hamstring injury, the Shoulder Bridge, because of its torso stabilizing movement, is excellent as a rehabilitation exercise.

Method (beginners)

- Lie on your back, knees bent, feet in line with the hips.
- Relax your arms down by your sides.

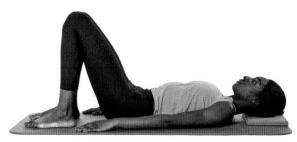

- Perform a few pelvic tilts to find your neutral spine and begin to activate those glutes.
- Engage your glutes (by squeezing) and engage your abdominal/pelvic floor muscles.
- Breathe in to your rib cage to prepare.

- Breathe out as you slowly curl from the base of your spine, off the floor, one vertebrae at a time towards the ceiling.

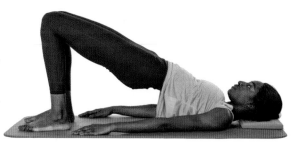

Breathe in at the top.
Breathe out as you gently and slowly lower your spine back down to the floor, one vertebrae at a time.
Repeat up to 10 times and then come into a full body stretch.

▶

Note
- Make sure your hips don't come higher than your knees when your spine is lifted off the floor – check that you have a straight line from knees to shoulders.
- Keep the weight evenly distributed between your feet.
- Be aware of any wobble – try to keep your torso steady throughout.
- Keep those abdominal and glute muscles engaged throughout.
- Concentrate on your breathing to help the exercise flow.

Progress (beginner/intermediate)

This progression of the Shoulder Bridge exercise challenges your coordination as well as improving shoulder mobility. If you choose to use light hand weights you will also be working your arms and increasing the challenge of keeping your torso stable.

- Lie on your back, knees bent, feet in line with the hips.
- Relax your arms down by your sides, with weights if you are using them.
- Perform a few pelvic tilts to find your neutral spine.
- Engage your glutes and abdominal/pelvic floor muscles.

- Breathe in to your rib cage to prepare.
- Breathe out as you lift both your arms, extending them backwards. At the same time slowly curl from the base of your spine, off the floor, one vertebrae at a time towards the ceiling.

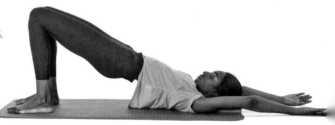

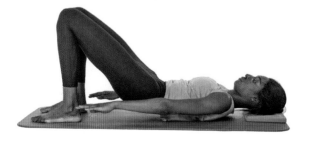

- Breathe in at the top.
- Breathe out as you simultaneously take your arms slowly back down to the mat while gently lowering your spine down to the floor.

- Repeat up to 10 times. When you have completed the repetitions and have come back down to the floor, bring both your knees into your chest and give them a hug.

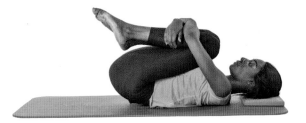

- Rotate your knees first one way and then the other, massaging your lower back, before coming into a full body stretch.

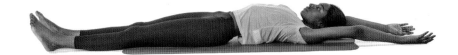

Progress (intermediate)

This progression of the Shoulder Bridge exercise has the added benefit of an abdominal curl included at the end. The coordination of this exercise is more challenging than the previous versions, so take the exercise slowly and try to keep the movements flowing.

Lie on your back, knees bent, feet in line with the hips. Relax your arms down by your sides, with weights if you are using them.

- Perform a few pelvic tilts to find your neutral spine.
- Engage your glutes and abdominal/pelvic floor muscles.
- Breathe in to your rib cage to prepare.
- Breathe out as you lift both your arms, extending them backwards. At the same time slowly curl from the base of your spine, off the floor, one vertebrae at a time towards the ceiling.

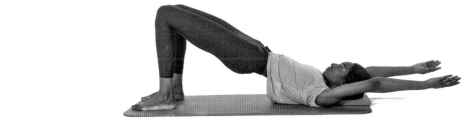

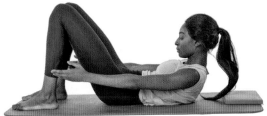

- Breathe in at the top.
- Breathe out as you simultaneously take your arms slowly back towards the mat and return your spine to the floor. When your glutes reach the mat, raise your head and neck and look towards your thighs.
- Breathe in as you hold the position.

▶

- Breathe out as your take your head back down to the floor and start to curl back up into the Shoulder Bridge position.
- Repeat up to 10 times. When you have completed the repetitions and have come back down to the floor, bring both your knees into your chest and give them a hug.

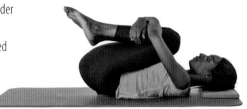

- Rotate your knees first one way and then the other, massaging your lower back, before coming into a full body stretch.

Progress (advanced)

This advanced version of the Shoulder Bridge exercise works those glute muscles even harder by increasing the pelvic stability challenge. It also targets all the core muscles.

- Lie on your back, knees bent, feet in line with the hips.
- Relax your arms down by your side with weights if you are using them.
- Perform a few pelvic tilts to find your neutral spine.

- Engage your glutes and abdominal/pelvic floor muscles.
- Breathe in to your rib cage to prepare.
- Breathe out as you slowly curl from the base of your spine, off the floor, one vertebrae at a time towards the ceiling.

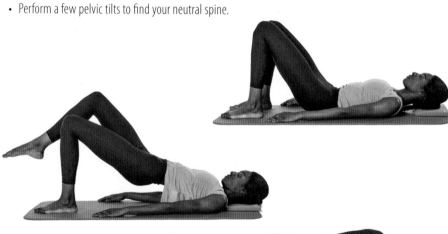

- Breathe naturally.
- In the raised Shoulder Bridge position lift your right foot off the floor.

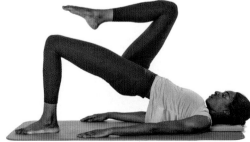

- Bend the knee towards your chest.

- Straighten the leg towards the ceiling, pointing your toes.
- Breathe in, holding that position.

- Breathe out and lower your raised leg to the same height as the bent knee.

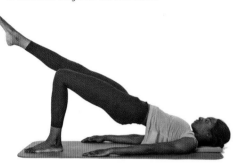
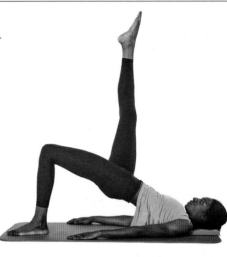

Breathe in and lift your right leg up to the ceiling, again keeping your hips stable.

Repeat 4 times.
Bend your knee back towards your chest and lower your right foot to the ground and then gently curl your spine back down to the floor.

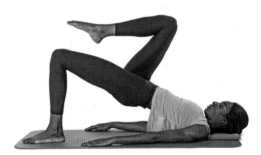

Repeat on the other side 4 times. Bring both your knees into your chest and hug them. Rotate first one way and then the other, massaging your lower back in the process. Come into a full body stretch.

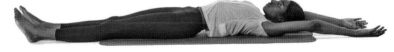

Note

- Keep your pelvis stable and hips level – if you notice that you are tilting to one side, lift the glute back up into the correct position.
- Be aware of torso stability and what the rest of your body is doing. Correct any wobbling that might be going on.

- Keep abdominal muscles and glutes engaged throughout.
- Sometimes this exercise can cause cramping in the hamstrings. This often happens if the glutes aren't being activated enough or are weak – as in running, the hamstrings take over! So make sure you are squeezing those buttock muscles.

SINGLE LEG BRIDGE (INTERMEDIATE/ADVANCED)

Running benefits

This is another development of the fantastic Shoulder Bridge, with the added challenge of performing the exercise one side at a time. As well as all the same running benefits of the full Shoulder Bridge, the Single Leg Bridge challenges stability and control of the pelvis even more and can show up any imbalances in the glutes and hip area. For example, you might find that one side feels stronger than the other as you perform the exercise, an indication that glute strength is unequal. Or you might find that on one side the hip flexors feel less comfortable.

Method

- Lie on your back, knees bent, feet in line with the hips.
- Relax your arms down by your sides.
- Come into neutral spine.
- Engage your abdominal muscles/pelvic floor muscles and glutes.
- Breathe in to prepare.
- Breathe out and gently peel your spine off the mat and into the Shoulder Bridge position (page 135).

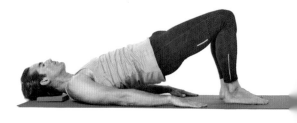

- Breathe in at the top.
- Breathe out and take your right foot off the floor, lengthening the leg to the ceiling and pointing your toe.

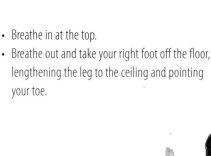

- Breathe in and lower your spine slowly and with control back down to the floor.

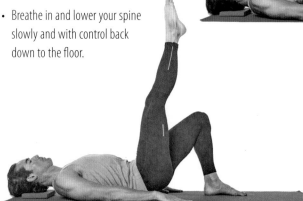

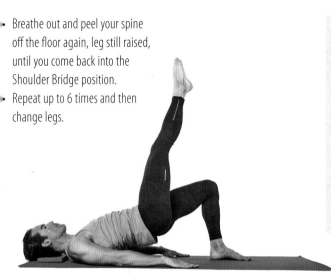

- Breathe out and peel your spine off the floor again, leg still raised, until you come back into the Shoulder Bridge position.
- Repeat up to 6 times and then change legs.

Note
- Make sure you keep your hips level.
- Keep your abdominal muscles and glutes engaged throughout.
- Concentrate on keeping the rest of the body relaxed and use your breathing to help the exercise to flow.

CASE STUDY

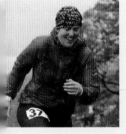

Lotty Bradford has run three marathons and loves off-road, trail and fell running.

I started practising Pilates over 12 years ago, long before I started running. I strongly believe though that building a strong core, stretching regularly and developing a much better awareness of my body and how it functions has all directly impacted on my ability to run and to remain injury-free. Pilates certainly helps me to stay upright! By having a strong core I'm able to cope with the demands of the unstable ground and foot placements. Pilates helped me with my recovery from a stroke too – I was only 28 but my balance was massively affected by it. Working on my Pilates helped improve that and means that I have the strength and confidence to run freely on the trails.

HIP CIRCLES (INTERMEDIATE/ADVANCED)

Running benefits

This exercise improves hip mobility, strengthens the hip flexors, the adductor muscles (inside thigh), the abductor muscles (outside thigh) and the core muscles. While circling the leg you'll be focused on hip and pelvis stability, which can be quite challenging but brings about an awareness of how easy it is for the pelvis to be unstable when running. This is also a good exercise for stretching those tight hamstrings.

Method

- Lie on your back, knees bent, feet in line with the hips.
- Come into neutral spine.
- Engage your abdominal/pelvic floor muscles.
- Raise your right leg and lengthen it to the ceiling, pointing your toes.

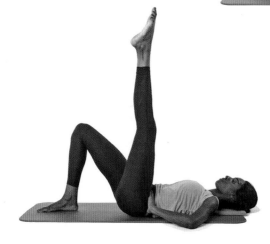

- Breathe in to your rib cage to prepare.
- Breathe out and, moving from the hip, draw small circles on the ceiling with your toes.
- Breathe in again, still circling the leg.
- Breathe out and reverse the movement, still keeping the circles small.
- Breathe in as you bring the leg back to centr

- Breathe out and sweep the leg around to the side of your body, extend down to the front and across your torso, making a big, wide circular movement.

- Repeat using your lateral thoracic breathing and moving on your outward breath for 4 rotations each side.
- Change sides.

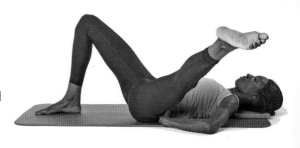

Note

- Place your hands on your hips so that you can feel any movement in the pelvis.
- Make sure your hip does not come off the floor as you rotate.
- The larger the circle the more challenging it will be, so be aware of your pelvic stability.

- Keep the movement flowing and smooth.
- If you find the pelvis moves around then keep the circles small to start with.
- Keep your abdominal muscles engaged and be aware of what the bent knee is doing.
- Is it flailing around and joining in? If so, stabilize!

Modify (beginners)

Use a Dyna-Band™ or yoga strap — hook the band around the sole of your left foot and hold the ends in your left hand.
Take your other arm out to the side to stabilize your torso.
Guide your leg around in a circle keeping the pelvis stable.
Repeat 4 times on each side.

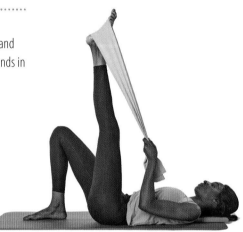

Progress (advanced)

Increase repetitions.
Draw larger circles but make sure the pelvis isn't joining in and that your abdominal muscles stay engaged.

> I love the Shoulder Bridge because it makes me feel that it opens out my back and lengthens the muscles. I also like Hip Circles because I believe these have really strengthened my legs and taught me about keeping my pelvis stable when I run.
>
> Janet Lee, recreational runner

REVERSE LEG PULL (INTERMEDIATE/ADVANCED)

Running benefits

This challenging exercise will improve your running posture and strengthen your core, lumbar spine, hips, arms, shoulders and glutes. It opens out the chest, stretching the pectoral muscles that can become tight during long runs and when fatigued, or if you spend your day hunched over a computer. It is also a wonderful exercise for stretching hip flexors, which can get very tired from all the repetitive leg lifting when we run. Your deltoid muscles (upper arm) will be strengthened as well, helping improve arm drive when running. It promotes stabilization in the shoulders and challenges spinal and pelvic stability.

Note: *if you have wrist problems, place your hands on a small cushion or omit this exercise.*

Method

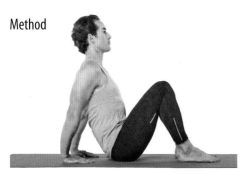

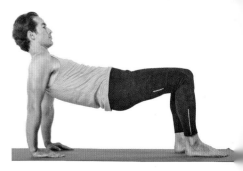

- Sit up tall on your 'sit bones' with your knees bent in front of you and feet flat on the floor.
- Place your hands directly behind your buttocks with your fingers facing towards your legs.

- Engage your abdominal/pelvic floor muscles.
- Breathe in to prepare.
- Breathe out and lift your torso off the ground into a box position.

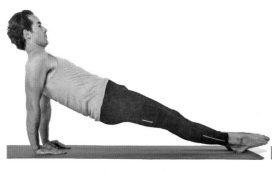

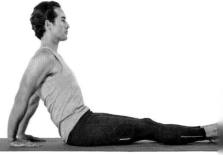

- Keep your head facing forwards, chin towards your chest.
- Breathe in and hold the position.
- Breathe out and lengthen first one leg and then the other leg out in front of you.

- Use your lateral thoracic breathing and hold for 3 breaths.
- Breathe in again.
- Breathe out and slowly lower yourself back down the floor with your legs still extended.
- Repeat 4 times and then come into a full body stretc

Note
- For some, the hand position can be uncomfortable. Change direction, pointing your fingers away from your body if you find that to be more comfortable.

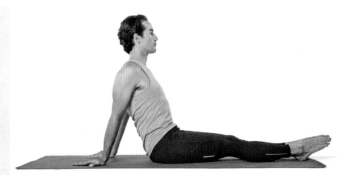

Modify (beginners)
- Perform fewer repetitions and hold for fewer breaths at the top.
- Complete the exercise after lifting into the start position, with bent knees/box shape only. Or just extend one leg at a time, returning to the bent knee position.

Keep the hips and chest open and your torso stable.
Concentrate on your breathing to help the exercise flow.

Progress (advanced)
Sit up tall on your 'sit bones' with your knees bent in front of you and feet flat on the floor. Place your hands directly behind your buttocks with your fingers facing towards your legs.

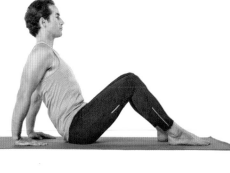

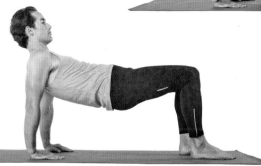

- Engage your abdominal/pelvic floor muscles.
- Breathe in to your rib cage to prepare.
- Breathe out and lift your torso off the ground into a box position.
- Keep your head facing forwards, chin towards your chest.

▶

- Breathe in and hold the position.
- Breathe out and lengthen first one leg and then the other leg out in front of you.
- Breathing naturally and from this extended leg position, quickly lift one leg up towards the ceiling, flexing your foot.

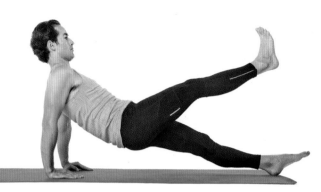

- Return it to the start position, pointing your toe.
- Repeat on the other side.
- Repeat 6 times in total and then bring your torso gently down to the floor and into a full body stretch.

Note

- As you become more confident with this progression, start to use the lateral thoracic breathing: breathe in when lifting the leg, breathe out when lowering it.

- Increase repetitions if you feel confident but keep your torso stable and chest open.
- Maintain a straight line from shoulders to toes; don't let your body sag.

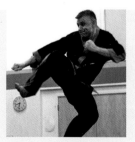

CASE STUDY

Graham Parkes, senior instructor at Bytomic Tae Kwon Do and a Black belt 5th Dan, has been running for three years. He runs mainly for health and fitness reasons and describes himself as a recreational runner. He attends a Pilates class once a week.

Pilates has taught me about muscle control, it focuses my mind on slower, more controlled movement and this benefit transfers not only to my running but also TKD which is a much more explosive form of exercise. Since practising Pilates I am more aware of what my body is doing and I'm definitely stronger. I've become a stronger runner well but it hasn't been easy, although that's probably a mental thing more than anything – coming to a Pilates class once a week and getting into the Pilates 'zone' clears my mind, and focusing on how my body moves really helps me to be more 'in my body'. I have to say that Pilates is really brilliant for the mind too!

SCISSORS (ALL LEVELS)

Running benefits

This exercise will give your hamstrings a really good stretch. It will also mobilize your hips while strengthening your core muscles, encouraging the torso to remain stable as you dynamically and rhythmically move your legs (as in running). It will also challenge your coordination, build stamina and stretch your upper back, improving your running posture.

Note: if your hamstrings are very tight, modify the exercise (however, if they are tight, they probably need a good stretch!).

Method

- Lie on your back.
- Bend both knees, feet in line with the hips.
- Come into neutral spine and make sure your body is relaxed with your arms down by your sides.
- Engage your abdominal/pelvic floor muscles.
- Raise your right leg and lengthen it to the ceiling, pointing your toes.

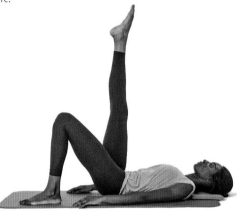

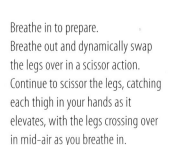

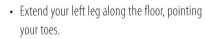

- Extend your left leg along the floor, pointing your toes.
- Curl your head and neck up and look towards your right knee.
- Wrap your hands lightly around the sides of your calf or thigh.

Breathe in to prepare.
Breathe out and dynamically swap the legs over in a scissor action. Continue to scissor the legs, catching each thigh in your hands as it elevates, with the legs crossing over in mid-air as you breathe in.

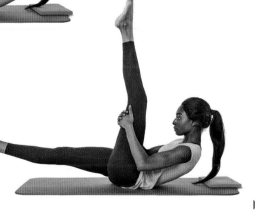

▶

- Keep your lower leg hovering above the floor – putting it down on the floor is cheating!
- Repeat for 16 scissors.
- Finish by lowering your head to the floor and bringing both knees into your chest. Then take one leg at a time down to the floor before coming into a full body stretch.

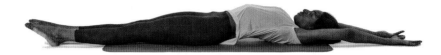

Note

- Keep the pelvis stable and spine in neutral while you move your legs. Slow the exercise down if you find your pelvis is moving so that you can concentrate on the all-important stability.

- Your hands should be lightly touching each leg. Don't pull the leg – your abdominal muscles should be doing the work and engaged throughout.
- If your hamstrings are tight, modify.

Modify

- If your hamstrings are very tight, bend your knees towards your chest a little.
- If you find you are tensing your neck muscles, put your head down and keep your arms by your sides. You can just move the legs and aim to improve the flexibility of the hamstrings while working on strengthening your core muscles.

- Keep in neutral spine, abdominals engaged throughout. Don't let your back arch – if it does then don't take your legs right down to the floor, let them hover halfway.

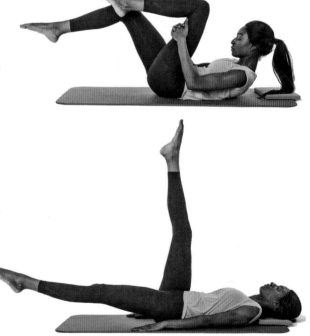

Progress

- Increase repetitions.
- Add a beat to the lower leg for the count of 2, but make sure the pelvis remains stable.

ROLLING LIKE A BALL (ALL LEVELS)

Running benefits

This exercise mobilizes the lumbar spine (page 27), often a tight part of the lower back post-run. It also massages and opens up all the back muscles, which can reduce any tension, and stretches the glutes. In addition, this exercise improves abdominal strength and coordination. There is also the opportunity to challenge your balance as you progress. You might have practised this exercise as a child, either on a trampoline or your own bed – it has a wonderful freeing feeling to it!

Note: if you have serious back problems or bone density problems, please omit this exercise.

Method

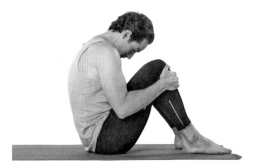

- Sit up tall on your 'sit bones' and, if you're using a mat, move yourself to the front edge so that you have space behind you to roll back. Please make sure you have moved any furniture out of the way around you because this is a dynamic exercise and it's quite easy to go off course when you first try it.
- Bend your knees, with feet flat on the floor.
- Rest your hands lightly on your shins and tuck your chin in to your chest.

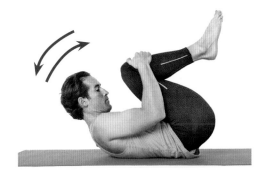

- Engage your abdominal/pelvic floor muscles.
- Breathe in to prepare.
- Breathe out and, with momentum, roll yourself backwards like a ball and then come straight back up again.

- Repeat 10 times and then come into a full body stretch.

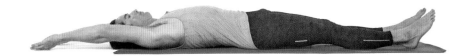

Note

- Make sure you keep your chin tucked in to your chest and that you don't roll back on to your neck.
- Keep the breathing going and make sure your abdominal muscles are engaged throughout.
- Try not to use your arms to pull yourself back up each time.

> Rolling Like a Ball is my favourite as it's such a fun exercise and brilliant for the core and spinal mobility.
>
> Sarah Sawyer, ultra marathon runner and Pilates instructor

Progress

- Increase repetitions.
- Perform the exercise slowly with less momentum, which will require more abdominal control.
- Challenge your balance by keeping your feet hovering above the floor when you return to the sitting position – stop the wobble by engaging those abdominal muscles!

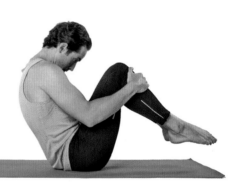

- Hold for longer at the top with your feet off the floor.

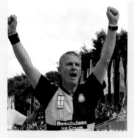

CASE STUDY

Mark Burrell only started running in 2012 and now runs trails, marathons and ultras, completing five marathons and four ultras in the last two years. He blogs under the title of Ultrabonkers.

I started doing Pilates because my physio was fed up with my hips and pelvis being out of line, she needed to straighten me up! Also to help running efficiency through better core strength, posture and speed.

Since then I've had fewer injuries as everything is working in line from glutes, hammys, quads, etc. I used to think I had 'runner's knee', but it was my hips, pelvis and glutes not working well, so not supporting my knee. My favourite exercise is the Shoulder Bridge as it helps my running form, and the various types of side lying exercises that particularly help my hip flexors, plus any moves that allow me to switch my glutes on.

ROLL BACK (BEGINNER)

Running benefits

This exercise strengthens the abdominal and hip muscles. It's also a good exercise to start with if you find the Roll Up (page 142) too challenging.

Method

- Sit up tall on your 'sit bones' and bend your knees, feet flat on the floor.
- Place your hands lightly around the sides of both thighs.

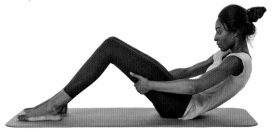

- Engage your abdominal/pelvic floor muscles.
- Breathe in to prepare.
- Breathe out and slowly begin to round your back into a 'C' shape, scooping out your abdominal muscles.
- Start to lower your lumbar spine, vertebrae by vertebrae, down towards the floor.
- Stop when you get to the point where you feel you might just drop back if you go any further.

- Breathe in and hold the lowered position.
- Breathe out and slowly start to return to sitting position.
- Repeat 8 times and then come into a full body stretch.

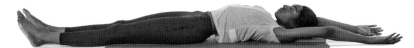

Note

- Imagine sending your ribs down towards your hips as you scoop out your abdominal muscles.
- Keep your abdominal muscles engaged and when you return to the sitting position, lengthen through your spine into a fully upright position.

Progress

Increase the repetitions.

Roll back with the aim of getting your spine closer to the floor.

Flex your feet as you perform the exercise for an added calf stretch.

Progress on to Roll Up with Spinal Stretch (page 142).

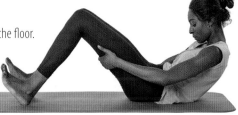

ROLL UP WITH SPINAL STRETCH (INTERMEDIATE/ADVANCED)

Running benefits

This exercise targets and strengthens the abdominal muscles and improves spinal and hamstring flexibility, which will increase your running power.

Method

- Lie on your back, legs extended in front of you.
- Engage your abdominal/pelvic floor muscles.
- Breathe in to prepare and raise your straight arms up above your chest.

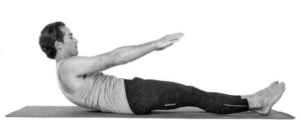

- Breathe out and start to curl your head, neck and torso up off the floor until you reach a tall sitting position.
- Breathe in at the top.

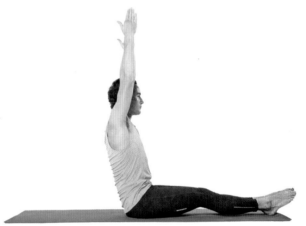

- Breathe out and lengthen yourself forwards, stretching your arms towards your feet into a spinal stretch.
- Breathe in as you hold the stretch.

- Breathe out and lift your arms up, sitting upright, and then gently roll yourself back down, with control, to the lying position.

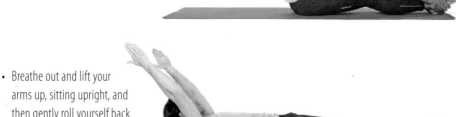

- Repeat 8 times. Come into a full body stretch.

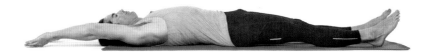

Note
- Keep the movement slow. Use your breathing to help the exercise flow and keep lengthening through the spine as you engage those abdominal muscles.
- Don't let your legs lift up off the floor.
- Make sure you return to the lying position in a slow, controlled manner; try not to flop back down to the floor with relief!

Modify
If your abdominal muscles aren't quite strong enough and you find it hard to get yourself off the floor without adding momentum, try rolling up a small towel and placing it underneath your lower back – sometimes this works, especially if you suffer from Lordosis (page 27).

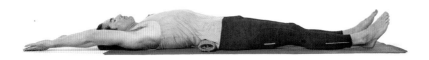

Try performing the exercise with your knees bent.

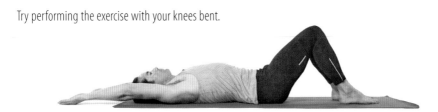

For beginners, try the Roll Up with Dyna-Band™ (page 144).

ROLL UP WITH DYNA-BAND™ (BEGINNER)

Method

- Sit up tall on your 'sit bones' and bend your knees.
- Take your Dyna-Band™, hook it around the soles of your feet and extend your legs out in front of you.
- Hold on tight to the ends of the Dyna-Band™.

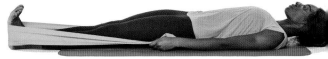

- Engage your abdominal/pelvic floor muscles.
- Breathe in to prepare.
- Breathe out and lower yourself gently down to the floor, scooping out your abdominal muscles as you do so.

- Breathe in when you reach the floor.
- Breathe out and use the Dyna-Band™ to gently lever yourself up off the mat slowly and with control, but make sure you aren't using your arms too much — those abdominal muscles need to work!

- Repeat up to 10 times.

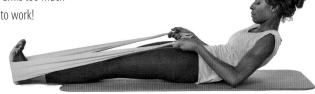

Note

- Keep your shoulders stabilized; try not to let them rise up around your ears when you are levering yourself up to the sitting position.
- Engage your abdominal muscles throughout.
- Concentrate on your breathing to help the exercise flow.

HIP TWIST WITH STRETCHED ARMS (ADVANCED)

Running benefits

This exercise opens up the chest, strengthens all the abdominal muscles including the oblique muscles, and strengthens the quads and hip flexors. The rotation and the stamina it demands will enhance your running performance. It teaches the torso to stay balanced and still while the legs are circling.

Note: if you have a back, wrist or elbow problem, please modify.

Method

- Sit up tall on your 'sit bones' and bend your knees, feet flat on the floor.
- Place your hands on the floor behind you, positioned slightly wider than your hips with your fingers facing backwards (or if you find it more comfortable, with your fingers facing outwards).
  Lean back and take your weight on to your hands.

Engage your abdominal/pelvic floor muscles. Raise one leg and lengthen it in front of you, pointing your toes.
Raise the other leg to join it, coming into a V position, legs together, toes still pointed.

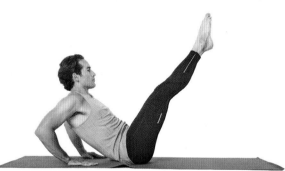

Breathe in to prepare.

Breathe out and slowly begin to circle your legs around to the right side of your body, continuing downwards and then to the other side.

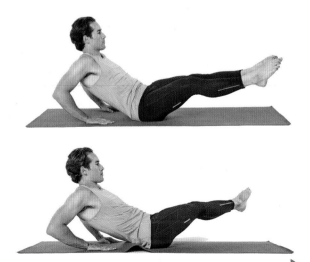

▶

- Breathe in as you return to the starting position.
- Repeat 4 times in one direction and then rotate 4 times the other way.
- Come into a full body stretch.

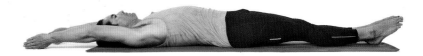

Note

- Try not to collapse in your centre. Keep lengthened and keep your abdominals engaged throughout, supporting your spine.
- Maintain torso and pelvic stability – don't let them join in and circle with your legs.

- Keep the exercise flowing and try to avoid jerky movements.
- Relax your shoulders; make sure they don't end up around your ears.
- Keep your legs straight, toes pointed and together.
- Breathe!

Modify

- Perform the exercise while leaning back on your forearms, elbows bent.

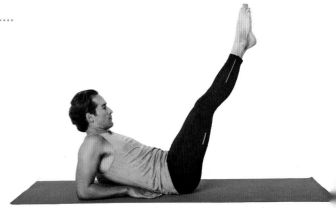

- Take your legs from side to side instead of in a full circle.

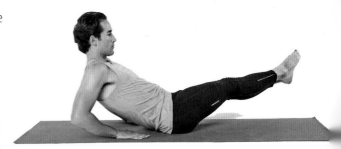

- If you attempt the rotations, keep them small until you feel confident that your pelvis isn't moving and your abdominal muscles feel stronger.

CRISS-CROSS (ALL LEVELS)

Running benefits

This exercise works the oblique muscles (waist), as do many of the Side Kick series (pages 88 to 94). By strengthening your oblique muscles you will find that there will be less side to side twisting in your running form. This twisting often occurs when the body is flagging towards the end of a long run and so wastes precious energy. In addition, this exercise is a great core strengthener: it works the lower abdominals, stretches the hip flexors, deep neck flexors, and it improves mobility of the thoracic spine (page 27). It will also improve coordination.

Note: if you have neck or back problems please take care or modify.

Method

- Lie on your back.
- Bend your knees, feet in line with your hips.
- Relax your arms down by your sides.
- Perform a few pelvic tilts to find your neutral spine position.
- Engage your abdominal/pelvic floor muscles.
- Raise your right leg up into the tabletop position.

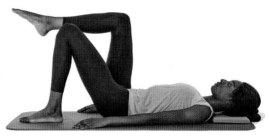

Raise your left leg up into the tabletop position.
Place your fingers lightly behind your head, taking your elbows out to the sides.
Raise your head and your neck off the floor and look towards your knees.

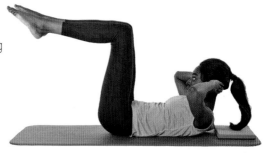

Breathe in to prepare.
Breathe out and rotate your torso to your left knee as you extend your right leg out in front of you, pointing your toes.

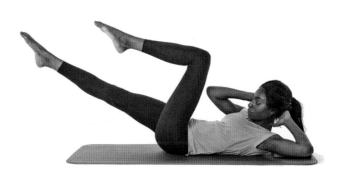

▶

- Breathe in as you return to centre.

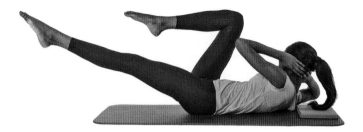

- Breathe out and rotate your torso to the other side, extending the opposite leg away.
- Repeat 2 sets of 10 repetitions, resting between each set of 10.
- At the end of the exercise lower your head and neck to the floor and bring your knees into your chest. Give them a hug before returning first one and then the other leg down to the floor. Come into a full body stretch.

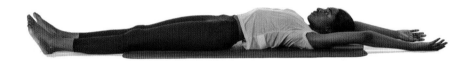

Note

- Keep your elbows relaxed and wide at the side of your head and be careful not to drag your head and neck forwards.
- Make sure your shoulders stay up off the floor throughout the exercise.

- Try to keep the movement flowing and use your breathing.
- Maintain pelvic stability and concentrate on keeping your abdominals engaged, extending your legs out in line with your hips.

Modify

- Perform fewer repetitions.
- Keep your feet on the floor with knees bent throughout the exercise. Curl up towards the knees and then rotate.

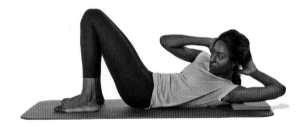

Progress

- Complete more repetitions.
- Take your legs lower to the ground when you extend, but be very careful that your back doesn't arch if you do so.

TEASER (ADVANCED)

Running benefits

This is a challenging but amazing exercise that benefits the runner in many ways. It strengthens all the core muscles – those abdominal muscles in particular will love you! It also strengthens the hip and neck flexors and enhances spinal mobility. In addition, the Teaser will improve your coordination and balance – you'll know when it has hit the spot, but don't cheat by using too much momentum!

Note: if you have lower back problems, please modify and perform the Half-Teaser which follows on page 151.

Method

- Lie on your back in a full body stretch.

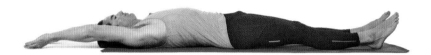

Engage your abdominal/pelvic floor muscles.
Breathe in to prepare.
Breathe out as you simultaneously lift your arms, legs and torso into a V shape, keeping your arms parallel with your legs.

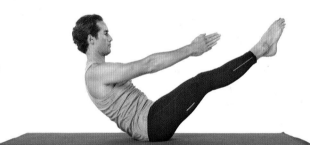

Breathe in as you balance steadily at the top.
Breathe out and slowly lower yourself back down to the floor with control, keeping your arms and legs coordinated and moving together as you roll back down.
Repeat up to 10 times and then come into a full body stretch.

Note

- This is one of the hardest Pilates exercises, so take care and start with a few repetitions before increasing.
- Make sure you keep your abdominal muscles engaged and your neck lengthened throughout the exercise.
- Try not to cheat by using too much momentum! Use your breathing to help keep the abdominal muscles activated and the movement controlled but flowing.

▶

Modify
- Perform the Half-Teaser instead (opposite).

Progress
- Increase the repetitions.
- When you are in the V position, lower your legs slightly – this will work your abdominal muscles even harder. Be careful not to arch your back.

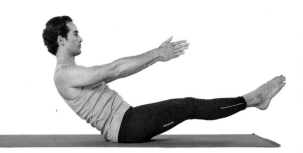

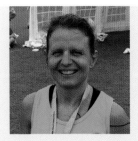

CASE STUDY

Tania Baldwin-Pask has been running for eight years and is a black belt in Tae Kwon Do. She attends Pilates classes once a week, as well as incorporating some of the exercises into her gym sessions and the warm ups that she runs at Tae Kwon Do.

Pilates has helped me to build a stronger, more stable core and this has impacted positively on my other sporting activities, particularly running. I used to unconsciously incorporate a lot of extra and unnecessary movement into my running – twisting at my waist a little as an extension of using my arms. Now I try to engage my core as I run an focus on powering through my legs, using my arms to help propel me forwards but without the twis. This is a much more efficient running style. When I trail run, particularly when it is muddy under-foot, I really notice that my core strength helps me stay on my feet. I've experienced pain in my groin/adductor muscles through an injury sustained two years ago and I sometimes find that engaging my pelvic floor helps keep this discomfort to a minimum. I notice that when I do my other sports that many sports people, regardless of age or gender, often struggle with their core strength. This has all sorts of implications for how they perform techniques, for efficiency and even for injury. I see Pilates a necessary foundation stone for any programme of exercise.

HALF-TEASER

This exercise is a modification of The Teaser on page 148.

Method

- Sit up tall on your 'sit bones' and bend your knees, feet flat on the floor.
- Take your weight on to your hands behind you, fingers pointing towards your legs.
- Engage your abdominal/pelvic floor muscles.
- Breathe in to prepare.
- Breathe out and raise your right leg diagonally up in front of you.

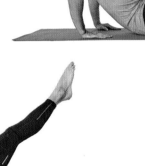

- Breathe in and hold that position.
- Breathe out and raise your left leg diagonally to join the right leg.

- Breathe in and hold the position.
- Breathe out and, bending your knee, lower one foot and then the other to the floor.
- Repeat up to 10 times and then come into a full body stretch.

Progress

When you are holding your legs in the V shape, take one hand off the floor and bring your arm forwards, parallel with your leg.

Eventually try to take both hands off the ground and hold the complete Teaser position (page 148).

Make sure you keep your abdominal muscles activated throughout the exercise. Practise this for a while until your abdominal muscles are stronger and you can progress on to the full Teaser.

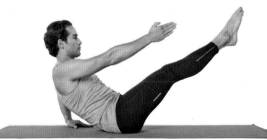

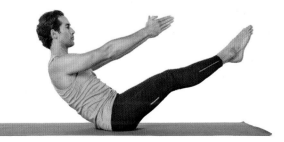

THE SAW (ALL LEVELS)

Running benefits

Like the Dart (page 64) and Swan Dive (page 60), this exercise will improve the mobility of the thoracic spine (page 27). When we run, this part of the back and shoulders can become tight as the muscles tire and the torso starts to collapse forwards. These muscles can also be affected by sitting hunched over a desk all day – I think I might have mentioned this several times before! The Saw will strengthen and stretch out those back muscles and the rotational movement in this exercise will strengthen the oblique muscles. You'll also feel a stretch in your hamstrings and adductor muscles.

Note: if you have disc problems, take care with this exercise and make sure rotation is comfortable.

Method

- Sit up tall on your 'sit bones' and come into neutral spine.
- Extend your legs out in front of you, placing them slightly wider than your shoulders.
- Flex your feet for a deeper stretch.
- Take your arms out to the sides of your body, level with your shoulders.

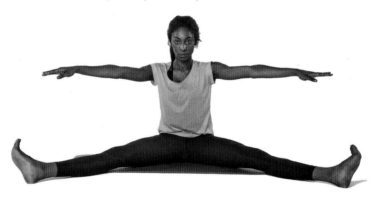

- Engage your abdominal/pelvic floor muscles.
- Breathe in to prepare and slowly rotate your torso to the right.

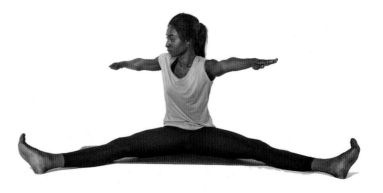

- Breathe out and, taking your chest down towards your leg, reach your left little finger towards your right little toe. Your right arm is lengthened behind your back.

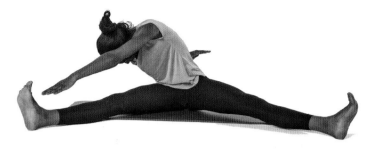

- Breathe in.
- Breathe out as you 'saw' your little finger three times towards and gently against your toe.
- Breathe in.
- Breathe out as you engage your abdominals to lift yourself back up to sitting, lengthening through the spine as you do so.
- Breathe in, sitting up tall again.
- Breathe out and repeat to the other side.

Repeat the exercise 3 times each side.

Note

- If you find your hamstrings or lower back are tight and sitting with your legs straight out in front of you is not possible, sit on a small cushion or block so that you can sit up tall and not collapse in your centre – this will improve the angle of your pelvis and increase mobility. Alternatively, modify the exercise.

Keep your abdominal muscles activated throughout.
Keep your knees and toes aligned, facing the ceiling, don't let your knees roll in.
Lift out of your hips as you rotate but make sure you don't rise up off the opposite buttock.

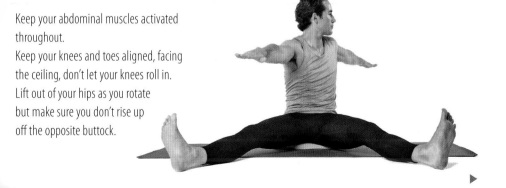

▶

Modify

- Bend your knees slightly if your hamstrings are really tight and bring your legs closer together.

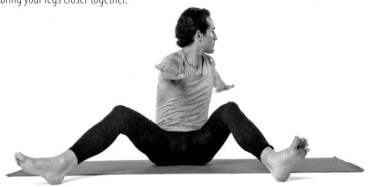

- If your shoulders or arms aren't comfortable being held out to the side, fold them in front of you and just rotate from side to side.
- Decrease repetitions.

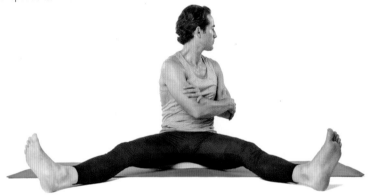

Progress

- Take your legs slightly wider apart but make sure you can still sit up on your 'sit bones' and the legs stay aligned.
- Increase repetitions.

For me personally having a strong core is equal to having a strong mind. Mine seem to be related! Also, I am quite a muscular build so it is important to keep my muscles lengthened.

Fleur Davey, recreational runner

PINE TWIST (ALL LEVELS)

nning benefits

s is a classic mat Pilates exercise that strengthens the obliques, abdominal and back muscles. It improves spinal bility, including the head and neck, but especially the thoracic spine (page 27). It's a great exercise to help prove running posture and the stability of your pelvis, but requires good abdominal control to keep the spine gthened and stable as you twist so that you remain sitting upright without slouching. This exercise is more allenging than it looks, so pay particular attention to your spinal alignment.

ote: if you have disc problems or a back injury, proceed with caution or omit this exercise.

ethod

Sit up tall on your 'sit bones' and come into neutral spine.
Extend your legs out in front of you along the floor with your feet flexed.
Take your arms out to the sides with your palms facing downwards.

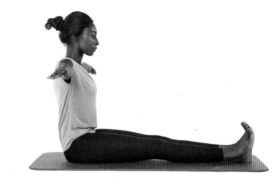

Engage your abdominal/pelvic floor muscles.
Breathe in to prepare as you lengthen through the spine.
Breathe out as you gently turn to the right and rotate your torso, starting with your head and neck and then through the rest of the spine until you are looking over your shoulder.

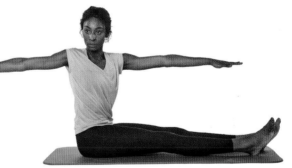

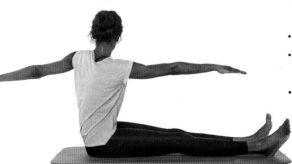

- Hold the position as you breathe in.
- Breathe out and return with control to centre.
- Repeat 5 times each side.

▶

Note

- Sitting upright on your 'sit bones' and staying in neutral position can sometimes be challenging, so sit on a small cushion or block to bring yourself into the correct position. Or modify the position that you sit in for the exercise.
- Make sure that you are rotating from your waist; engage those abdominals as you move so that your arms just move freely with you – don't use your arms to lead.
- Be aware of any movement in the pelvis and stabilize.

- Try not to lean forwards as you twist – your legs should remain still.
- Are your shoulders stabilized or are they coming up around your ears as you move?

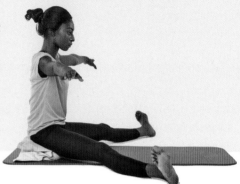

Modify

- If sitting with your legs out in front of you and remaining lengthened through the spine while maintaining a neutral position is challenging, or your hamstrings are so tight that you can't straighten your legs, choose one of the following leg positions:

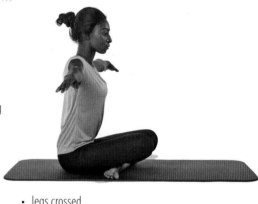

- legs crossed.

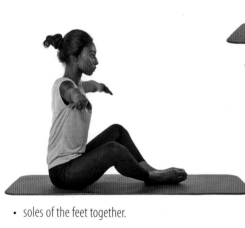

- soles of the feet together.

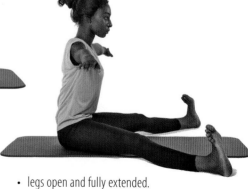

- legs open and fully extended.

- For shoulder problems that make holding your arms out to your sides uncomfortable, place your hands on your shoulders as you twist.

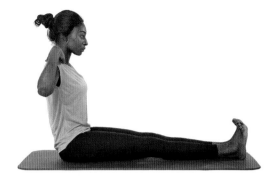

- Or bring your hands together in front of you into a praying position, elbows to the side.

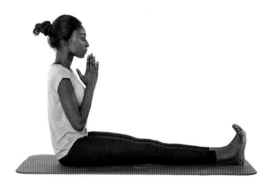

Alternatively, take your arms to the sides, fingertips/hands to the floor.

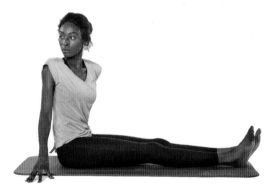

rogress
Increase repetitions.
Increase range of movement.

> Pilates has really kept me injury-free. I have some weak and tight muscles around my pelvis, which, if left unchecked, cause hip problems. Regular Pilates keeps my pelvis balanced and core strengthened. I love any Pilates exercise which works on my hips and butt!
>
> Fleur Davey, recreational runner

SPINAL MOBILITY AND OBLIQUE STRETCH (ALL LEVELS)

Running benefits

Although primarily a stretch, this exercise will strengthen the oblique muscles and so reduce any twisting in your torso as you run, which, as mentioned before, wastes precious running energy. This exercise is wonderful for the lower back and can be performed as part of your exercise routine or as a post-run stretch to relieve any lower back tension.

Method

• Lie on your back with your knees bent, feet in line with your hips and your arms stretched out by your sides.

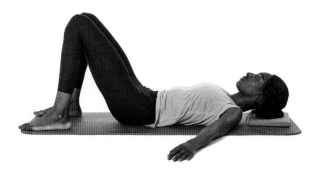

• Perform a few pelvic tilts to come into neutral spine.
• Engage your abdominal/pelvic floor muscles.
• Lift your right foot off the floor and inwardly rotate to place your right ankle across your left thigh.

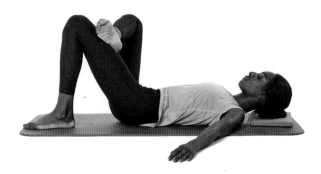

• Breathe in to prepare.

- Breathe out and let your right knee gently drop down to the floor, lifting your left hip as you do so and rotating in the spine.

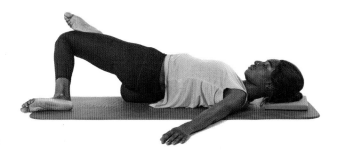

- Breathe in as you hold the stretch.
- Breathe out, engaging your abdominal muscles as you lift the knee back up to the start position.
- Repeat 4 times in total and then change sides.

Note
- Take your knee just halfway if you find the stretch too intense.
- Your opposite hip will lift off the floor, but keep the opposite shoulder down on the floor, don't let it join in.

The thing about Pilates is the way in which it makes you so aware of your posture and core, and from my perspective this is one of the things that's been most beneficial to my running. The increase in my core strength has made me a stronger runner. The other thing that has been beneficial is my teacher's comments on my strength and flexibility. For example, other than Pilates I do very little else other than run, and while I'm quite fit and my legs are quite strong, my teacher pointed out how inflexible my hip flexors are and I really work at the exercises to try and increase my flexibility. The other things that have been very useful are the balance exercises and these have strengthened my legs. My favourite exercise is probably the Plank and I actually try to do this daily. I also try and do the balance exercises a few times a week.

Sue Cunningham, marathon runner (retired!)

HIP ROLLS (ALL LEVELS)

Running benefits

A great exercise post-run or during your exercise routine to relieve tension in a tight lower back, it helps realign the spine and challenges the abdominal muscles and the obliques. The progression of this exercise also stretches out the hamstrings and calf muscles.

Method

- Lie on your back with your knees bent, legs and feet together.
- Take your arms out to the sides, placed just below shoulder level.

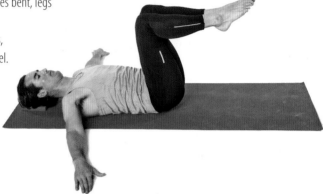

- Engage your abdominal/pelvic floor muscles.
- Breathe in to prepare.
- Breathe out and drop both your knees towards the floor on your right-hand side.
- Breathe in and hold the position.

- Breathe out as you return them back to centre.
- Repeat on the other side.
- Repeat 4 times each side.

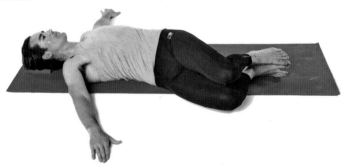

Note

- Try to keep the opposite shoulder on the mat.
- Keep your knees and legs connected throughout the exercise.

- Make sure you're using your abdominal muscles and not your back muscles when you lift your knees up off the floor – you will feel the difference.

Progress

- For a deeper stretch and spinal rotation, lift both your feet off the floor, knees over hips and shins parallel to the ceiling.
- Keep your legs and feet together and point your toes.
- Take your arms to the sides, placed just below your shoulders.
- Engage your abdominal/pelvic floor muscles.
- Breathe in to prepare.
- Breathe out and slowly lower both your knees to your right-hand side, with control, to the floor.

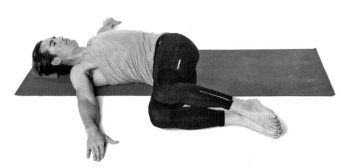

Now extend and lengthen the top leg along the still bent bottom leg.

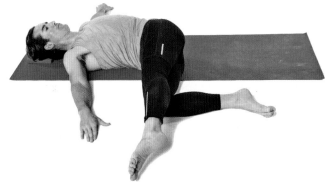

Hold the position for a couple of breaths.
Breathe in and slowly bend the knee back.

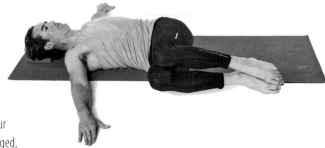

Breathe out and, making sure your abdominal muscles are still engaged, lift both knees back to centre.
Repeat 2 times to both sides.

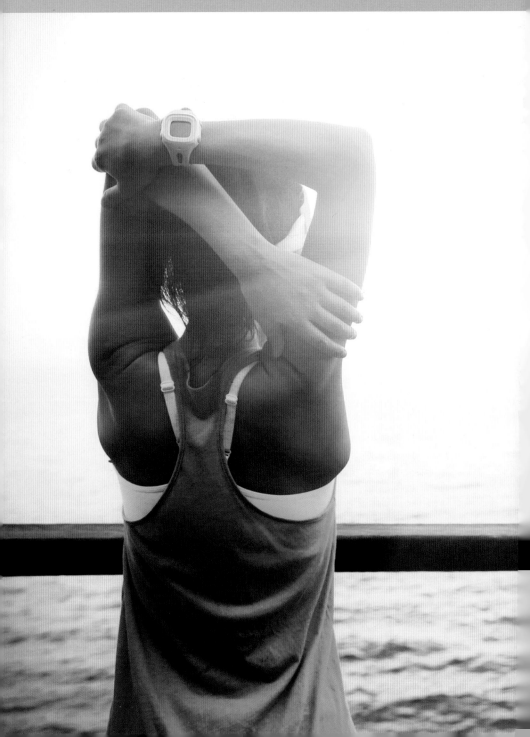

Chapter 8

Post-run stretches

The following stretches should be performed once the body is warmed up after a run, or at the end of your Pilates session. They feature a mixture of stretching techniques, some using a Dyna-Band™ which can be performed on a mat at home, and some standing. The standing stretches are more suitable for when you've come to the end of your run – or even during the run if you feel any muscle tightness.

- Aim to hold the stretch for approximately 20–30 seconds.

- Work within your ability, don't force a stretch.

- Only stretch to a point of mild tension, not to pain.

- Stretch slowly.

Note: *do not stretch in the first 24–72 hours following an injury, especially if caused by a fall or some kind of trauma. Seek specialist advice if in doubt. Do not bounce in the stretch.*

HAMSTRING, ADDUCTOR AND ABDUCTOR STRETCH WITH DYNA-BAND™

Method

Lie on your back with knees bent.
Extend your right leg up above your body and hook the centre of your Dyna-Band™ around the sole of your foot.
Hold one end of the Dyna-Band™ in each hand.
Engage your abdominal/pelvic floor muscles.
Breathe in to prepare.
Breathe out as you gently ease your right leg towards your head, feeling a gentle lengthening of the muscles in the back of your thigh.

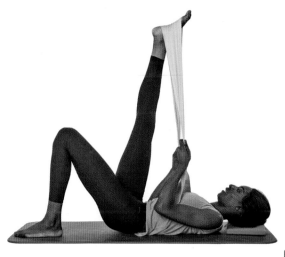

▶

- Breathe naturally and hold for 20–30 seconds.
- Release the stretch and then repeat a couple more times.
- Breathe in.
- Breathe out as you drop your right leg to the side – only take it to a comfortable position until you feel the gentle stretch on the inside of the thigh.

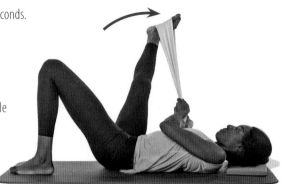

- Breathe naturally and hold the stretch for 20–30 seconds.
- Breathe in.
- Breathe out and lift the leg back up above your body then let it drop down across the other side of your torso so that you feel a stretch on the outside of the thigh. You might find that you don't have to take it very far to feel the stretch.

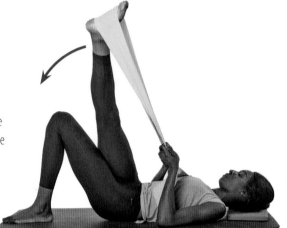

- Hold the stretch, breathing naturally for 20–30 seconds.
- Breathe in.
- Breathe out and raise the leg back up to centre.
- Change legs and repeat the whole stretching sequence from the beginning.

GLUTE/PIRIFORMIS STRETCH

Method

- Lie on your back with knees bent.
- Place your right ankle across your left thigh.
- Take your right hand between both legs and place it round the inside of your left thigh.
- Place your left hand around the outside of your left thigh.
- Engage your abdominal/pelvic floor muscles.
- Raise your head and neck off the floor and look towards your knees.
- Breathe in to prepare.
- Breathe out and slowly pull your left leg towards your chest as you feel a stretch in the buttock area.

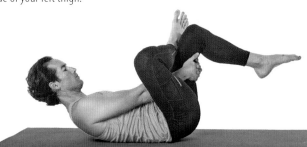

- Breathe naturally and hold the stretch for 20–30 seconds, then release.
- Repeat on the other side.

LYING QUAD STRETCH

Note: if you have problems with your knees, please take care.

Method

Lie on your side. Come up on to your elbow and support your head with your hand.

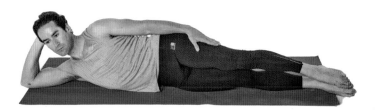

Bend your top knee as you breathe in. Breathe out and reach behind to take hold of your top foot or shin in your other hand. Gently ease your leg towards your glute.

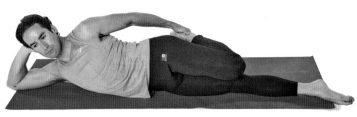

Breathe naturally and hold the stretch for 20–30 seconds. Repeat on the other side.

STANDING STRETCHES

CALF MUSCLE AND ACHILLES STRETCH

Method

- Stand tall and take your right leg behind you, pressing your heel into the ground.
- Bend your front knee, leaning forwards slightly but keeping your back straight.
- Hold for 20–30 seconds as you feel a lengthening in the back of your calf muscle.

- Change legs and repeat.

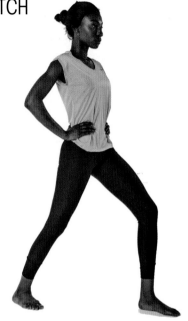

QUADRICEPS AND HIP FLEXOR STRETCH

Method

- Stand tall, engage your abdominal muscles and raise your right foot behind you towards your right buttock.
- Take hold of your ankle with your right hand.
- Gently ease your foot and leg with your hand towards your buttock until you feel a gentle stretch in the front of your thigh.

- If you find it hard to balance, hold on to something.
- Try not to arch your back.
- Take both knees together and tilt your pelvis back for a stronger stretch.

- Hold for 20–30 seconds, breathing naturally, and then change legs.

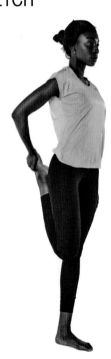

ITB STRETCH

Method

- Stand with your right leg crossed behind your left leg.
- Lean to your left but push your right hip out to the side.
- Bend your left knee slightly and keep your right leg straight.

- Hold for 30 seconds as you gently stretch out the ITB – you'll feel the lengthening from your right hip down to your right knee.
- Repeat on the other leg.

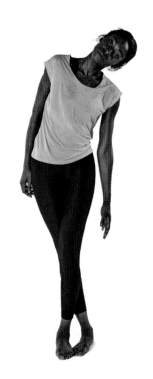

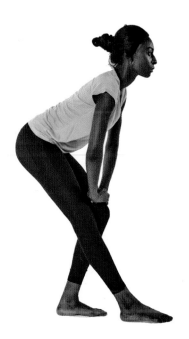

HAMSTRING STRETCH

Method

- Extend your right leg in front of your left – make sure both knees are parallel.
- Keep your right leg straight and bend your left knee.
- Place your hands on your left thigh for support and make sure you can feel the stretch at the back of your thigh.

- Hold for 20–30 seconds.
- Repeat on the other leg.

ADDUCTOR STRETCH

Method

- Standing tall, place your legs wide apart with feet parallel.
- Bend your right knee and make sure your knee stays over your foot, don't let it go beyond.

- Keep your left leg extended.
- Hold the stretch for 20–30 seconds and then change legs.

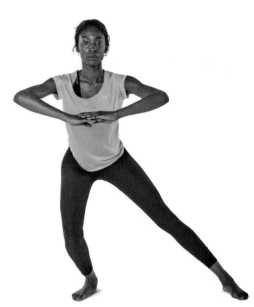

UPPER BACK AND CHEST STRETCH

Method

- Stand tall.
- Raise your arms in front of your chest and 'hug a tree'!

- Hold for about 20 seconds.

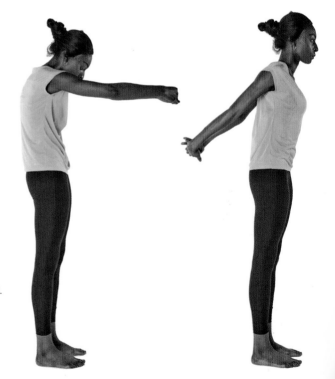

- Take your arms behind your back.
- Interlock your fingers and gently raise your arms upwards.

- Hold for about 20 seconds.

In addition, you could add the following Pilates exercises into your post-run stretching routine:

Roll Down (page 53)

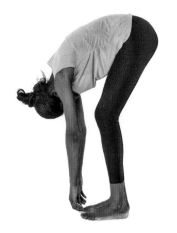

> The Roll Down is an exercise I now regularly use, pre- and post-runs. Just two or three seem to help and only take a few minutes.
>
> Paul Buckle,
> ultra runner

Cat Stretch (page 82)

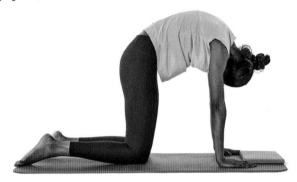

Chest Opener (page 103)

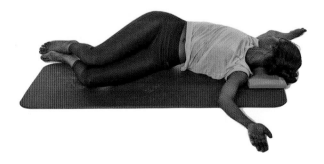

Extended Child's Pose (page 85)

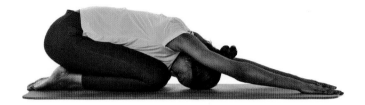

Cobra Stretch (page 87)

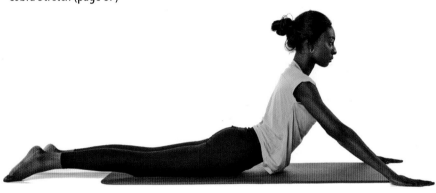

Hip Rolls (page 160)

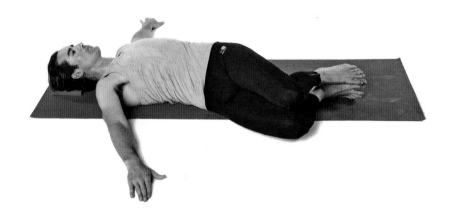

Spinal Mobility and Oblique Stretch (page 158)

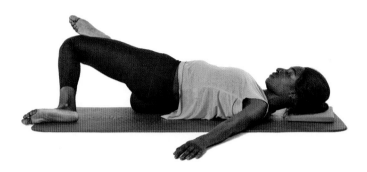

Shoulder Bridge (page 125)

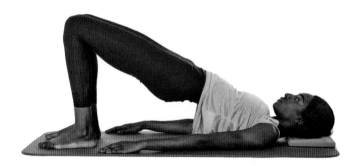

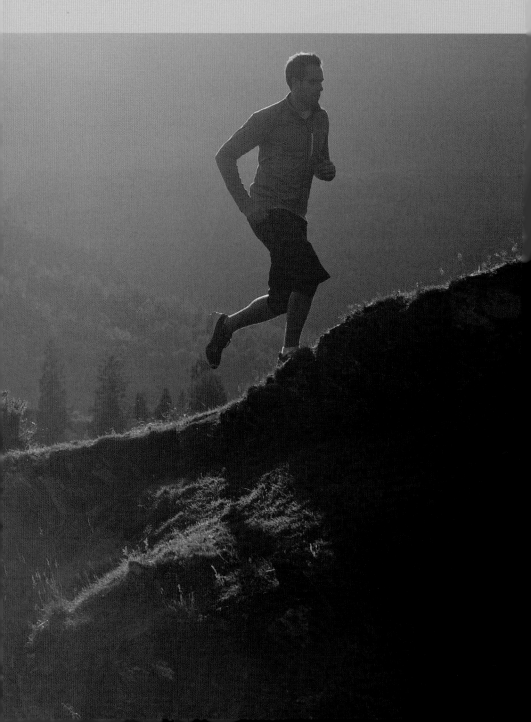

Chapter 9

Five 10–15-minute daily routines to improve your running

Practising some mat Pilates for just 15 minutes a day, or even every other day, will pay dividends in the long run. Take a look at the following exercises – these are suggested routines to get you into the habit of regular Pilates practice. If you're not sure which level to begin with, just start at the beginning – you'll soon discover what works for you and what needs improvement! But please do perform a warm up beforehand if you're doing these exercises pre-run, and you should ideally include some balancing as well. As you progress you will want to increase repetitions and maybe add or swap some of the exercises around depending on your needs, familiarity with the movements and time available. These routines will take you around 10–15 minutes to perform, but will obviously take a lot longer to begin with as you get to know the routines and need to refer back to the relevant page for instructions.

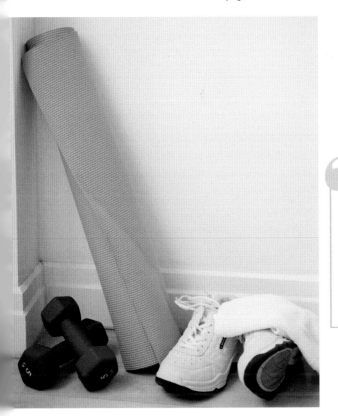

> Make up your mind that you will perform your Pilates exercises for 10 minutes without fail.
>
> Joseph Pilates

Beginner

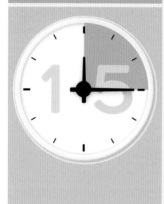

Day 1

Roll Down × 3 (page 53)

Swimming into Back Extension: 4 × 10 paddles, plus 2 Back Extensions (page 66)

Leg Pull Front / Plank (page 69)

Extended Child's Pose (page 85)

Side Kick 1 × 10 each side (page 86)

Clam: up to 16 each side (page 98)

Single Knee Folds × 4 each side (page 104)

Neck Curl Ups × 6 (page 115)

Shoulder Bridge × 8 (page 125)

Roll Back × 8 (page 141)

Rolling Like A Ball × 8 (page 139)

Hip Rolls × 2 each side (page 160)

Full Body Stretch

Day 2

Roll Down × 3 (page 53)

Ankle Mobility × 6 each way, plus 6 × point and flex (page 107)

Single Knee Folds × 4 each side (page 104)

The Hundred (preparation) × 2 (page 116)

The Hundred (page 118)

Shoulder Bridge, plus progression with arms × 8 (page 126)

Side Kick 2 + Inner Thigh × 10 each side (page 90)

Chest Opener × 6 each side (page 103)

Superman × 5 each side (page 62)

Extended Child's Pose (page 85)

Day 3

Roll Down × 1 (page 53)

Push Up from Standing: 2 sets × 3 Push Ups (page 78)

Swan Dive × 6 (page 60)

Outer and Inner Thigh Lifts × 16 each side (page 99)

Single Leg Stretch: aim for 20 in total, alternating legs (page 120)

Hip Circles with Dyna-Band™ × 4 rotations each way and with both legs (page 133)

Roll Up with Dyna-Band™ × 6 (page 144)

Spine Twist × 3 each side (page 155)

Full Body Stretch

Day 4

Roll Down × 3 (page 53)

Dart with Triceps × 6 (page 64)

Cat Stretch (page 82)

Single Leg Kick × 8 in total alternating legs (page 74)

Side Kick 1 × 10 each side (page 86)

Clam: up to 16 on each side (page 98)

Neck Curl Ups × 6 (page 115)

Single Knee Folds × 4 each side (page 104)

Scissors: up to 16 in total, alternating legs (page 137)

Rolling Like A Ball × 10 (page 139)

Criss-Cross × 10 (page 147)

Full Body Stretch

Day 5

Roll Down × 3 (page 53)

Shoulder Stability, plus Arm Circles × 6 of each (page 108)

Single Knee Folds × 4 each side (page 104)

Dead Bug × 8 each side (page 113)

Half-Teaser × 6 (page 151)

Side Kick 2 + Inner Thigh × 10 each side (page 90)

Rotational Cat × 6 each side (page 72)

Leg Pull Front / Plank, modify 2 version (page 69)

Extended Child's Pose (page 85)

Intermediate

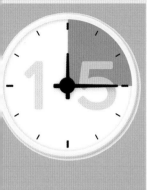

Day 1

Roll Down × 3 (page 53)

Swimming into Back Extension: 4 × 10 paddles, plus 4 Back Extensions (page 66)

Leg Pull Front / Plank, modify 1 version (page 69)

Extended Child's Pose (page 85)

Side Kick 1 × 10 each side (page 86)

Clam × 16 each side (page 96)

Single Knee Folds × 4 each side (page 104)

Neck Curl Ups × 6 (page 115)

Single Leg Stretch: aim for 20 in total, alternating legs (page 120)

Shoulder Bridge × 10 (page 125)

Hip Rolls × 2 each side (page 60)

Full Body Stretch

Day 2

Roll Down × 3 (page 53)

Ankle Mobility × 6 each way, plus 6 × point and flex (page 107)

Double Knee Fold × 6 in total, alternating legs (page 105)

The Hundred (preparation) × 2 (page 116)

The Hundred (page 118)

Shoulder Bridge (intermediate) × 6 (page 127)

Side Kick 2 + Inner Thigh × 10 each side (page 90)

Chest Opener × 6 each side (page 103)

Superman × 5 each side (page 62)

Extended Child's Pose (page 85)

Day 3

Roll Down × 1 (page 53)

Push Up from Standing – 2 sets × 3 Push Ups (page 78)

Swan Dive × 6 (page 60)

Cat Stretch (page 82)

Outer and Inner Thigh Lifts × 16 both sides (page 99)

The Hundred (preparation) × 2 (page 116)

Double Leg Stretch × 10 (page 122)

Hip Circles × 4 each way on both sides (page 132)

Roll Up, plus Spinal Stretch × 8 (page 142)

Spine Twist × 3 each side (page 155)

Full Body Stretch

Day 4

Roll Down × 1 (page 53)

Dart with Triceps plus weights (optional) × 4 reps with weights (6 without) (page 64)

Double Leg Kick × 6 (page 76)

Cat Stretch (page 82)

Side Kick 3 into Torpedo x 10 on both sides (page 92)

The Hundred (preparation) × 2 (page 116)

Scissors x 16 in total, alternating legs (page 137)

Single Leg Bridge × 3 each side (page 130)

Rolling Like A Ball × 10 (page 139)

Criss-Cross × 10 in total, alternating elbow to knee (page 147)

Full Body Stretch

Day 5

Roll Down × 3 (page 53)

Shoulder Stability, plus Arm Circles × 6 of each (page 108)

Single Knee Fold × 4 each side (page 104)

Dead Bug with weights (optional) × 8 each side (page 113)

Reverse Leg Pull × 4 (page 134)

Teaser × 6 (page 149)

Side Kick 4, plus hamstring × 10 on both sides (page 94)

Rotational Cat × 6 each side (page 72)

Leg Pull Front / Plank (page 69)

Extended Child's Pose (page 85)

Advanced

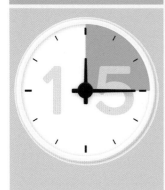

Day 1

Roll Down × 3 (page 53)

Swimming into Back Extension: 4 × 10 paddles, 4 Back Extensions (page 66)

Front Leg Pull / Plank × 6 leg raises in total alternating legs (page 69)

Side Kick 3 into Torpedo using hand weights (optional) × 10 on both sides (page 92)

Clam, feet lifted × 10 on each side (page 98)

Single Knee Fold × 4 each side (page 104)

The Hundred (preparation) × 2 (page 116)

The Hundred, legs extended (page 119)

Shoulder Bridge × 10 (page 125)

Hip Rolls × 2 each side (page 160)

Full Body Stretch

Day 2

Roll Down into Push Up from Standing × 3 with 3 Push Ups each time (page 78)

Ankle Mobility × 6 each way, plus 6 × point and flex (page 107)

Double Knee Fold × 8 in total, alternating legs (page 105)

The Hundred (preparation) × 2 (page 116)

Double Leg Stretch × 10 (page 122)

Shoulder Bridge (advanced) × 4 each side (page 129)

Side Kick 2, plus inner thigh × 10 each side (page 90)

Chest Opener × 6 each side (page 103)

Superman × 10 (page 62)

Extended Child's Pose (page 85)

The Saw × 3 each side (page 153)

Day 3

Roll Down × 3 with progressions (page 53)

Dart with triceps plus weights × 6 (page 64)

Outer and Inner Thigh Lifts × 16 each side (page 99)

The Hundred (preparation) × 2 (page 116)

The Hundred, legs extended (page 119)

Hip Circles × 4 each way on both sides (page 132)

Roll Up, plus Spinal Stretch × 10 (page 142)

Reverse Leg Pull × 6 with 3 Leg Raises each side (page 134)

Spine Twist × 3 each side (page 155)

Full Body Stretch

Day 4

Roll Down × 1 (page 53)

Swan Dive × 8 (page 60)

Cat Stretch into Down Dog (page 83)

Double Leg Kick × 8 (page 76)

Side Bend × 4, plus 'thread the needle' each side (page 96)

Clam, feet lifted × 10 and pulse × 10 each side (page 89)

Scissors × 16 in total, alternating legs (page 137)

Single Leg Bridge × 3 on each leg (page 130)

Rolling Like A Ball × 10 feet off the floor (page 139)

Hip Twist with stretched arms × 4 each way (page 145)

Full Body Stretch

Day 5

Roll Down × 3 (page 53)

Shoulder Stability, plus Arm Circles with weights × 4 of each (page 108)

Double Knee Fold × 4 each side (page 105)

Dead Bug with weights × 4 each side (page 113)

Criss-Cross × 10 alternating elbow to knee (page 147)

Teaser × 10 (page 149)

Side Kick 4 + Hamstring Stretch × 10 each side (page 94)

Rotational Cat × 6 each side (page 72)

Front Leg Pull / Plank (page 69)

Cobra Stretch (page 87)

Extended Child's Pose (page 85)

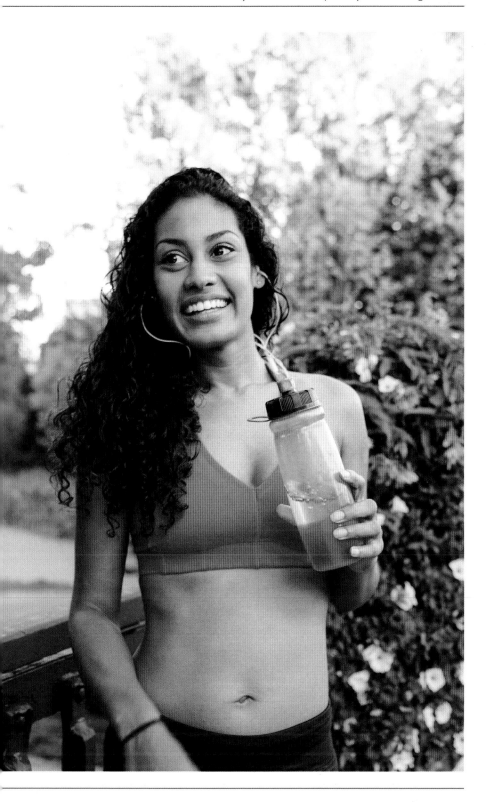

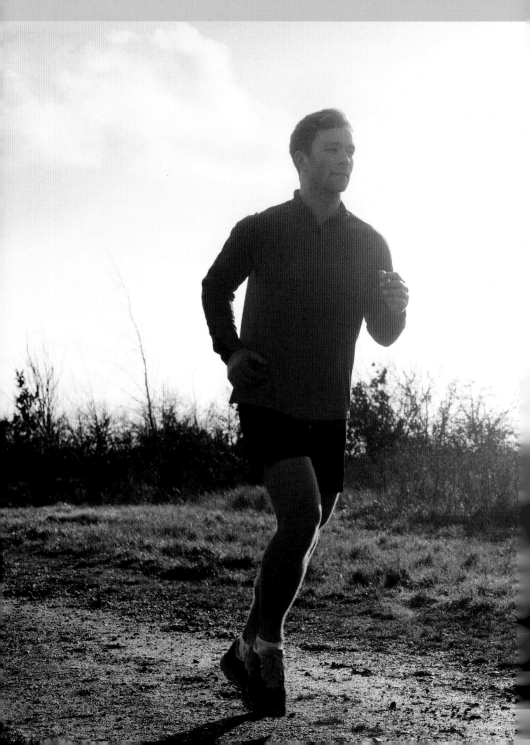

Chapter 10

The healing power of Pilates

Running can be a life-enhancing experience, whether you're a beginner just starting out on your running adventure or an ultra marathon runner. But runners are renowned for overdoing it and even developing an addiction to the sport. Sometimes the focus on training can become an obsession, to the point of disrupting further fitness, health or life in general. Sadly, there's a fine line between optimal training and overtraining.

There comes a time when no matter how hard you train, fitness levels or running performance just don't improve. In fact sometimes the opposite can happen. The 10k that once felt comfortable, now, no matter how much training you're putting in, becomes a huge effort. Research has shown that more than half of all runners will go through this and hit an overtraining plateau at some point in their running career. If you're constantly catching colds, finding it hard to sleep well, have lost your appetite and feel exhausted all the time, stop for a minute and think about whether you've been overtraining and are heading for burn out. Quite often it will be a member of your family who will notice it before you do.

Pilates exercises can provide a calm and healing down-time. They'll allow you to take stock, rest and give your body and mind the time and resources to recover, so that you can get back out there and run. But first comes the hardest part: you need to acknowledge that you've been overtraining.

Common symptoms of overtraining include:
- lack of appetite and weight loss
- sugar and caffeine cravings
- insomnia or interrupted sleep patterns
- frequent coughs, colds, headaches, sore throats and minor infections that just won't go away
- lack of sex drive
- minor injuries that take forever to heal
- depression, mood swings, irritability, loss of confidence
- heavy, achy legs or stiffness that just won't shift
- lack of concentration
- increase in resting heart rate.

The wonderful thing about Pilates is that it puts you in much closer touch with how your body is feeling and functioning. You'll begin to be more aware of minor changes, both mental and physical, during your training, in a way that you weren't before. As you learn to concentrate and perform the movements in the exercises and get to know your body better, you'll be surprised at how beneficial this form of body conditioning can be on every level.

An additional way to avoid overtraining would be to keep a journal of your runs – not just writing down your running times and route but also the regular Pilates sessions you're including and how you feel in general. A pattern might emerge of 'heavy legs', 'exhausted' or 'fed up', for example. This way you'll recognize the overtraining warning signs before you reach that tipping point and will be able to rein yourself in before the symptoms get out of hand.

I had always been a very traditional runner. My approach to training was more miles, and if in doubt more miles still. In 2013 at the age of 47 I ran a PB at 5k, 5 miles, 10k, 10 miles, half marathon, 20 miles and marathon, off the back of 80–90 miles a week. The result of this: a stress fracture of the pelvis that had me not running a step for eight months. As part of the long road to recovery I was persuaded to try Pilates. I found it has improved all areas of my running, and most importantly I run injury-free. I should also add that since starting Pilates my long-term back and knee problems have also been resolved. When I leave my classes, I feel taller, stronger and ready to run! I do classes/sessions at home 3–4 times a week, and now given a choice between missing a run or Pilates, the running would go.

Robin McCoy, marathon runner

Chapter 11

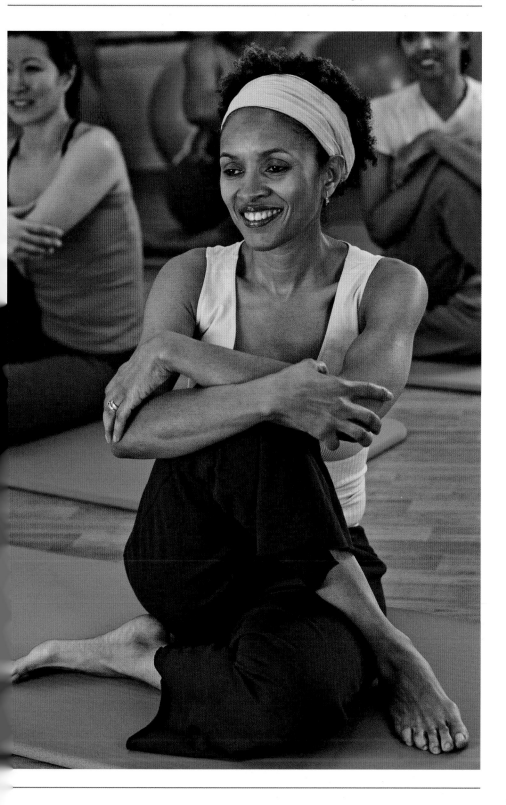

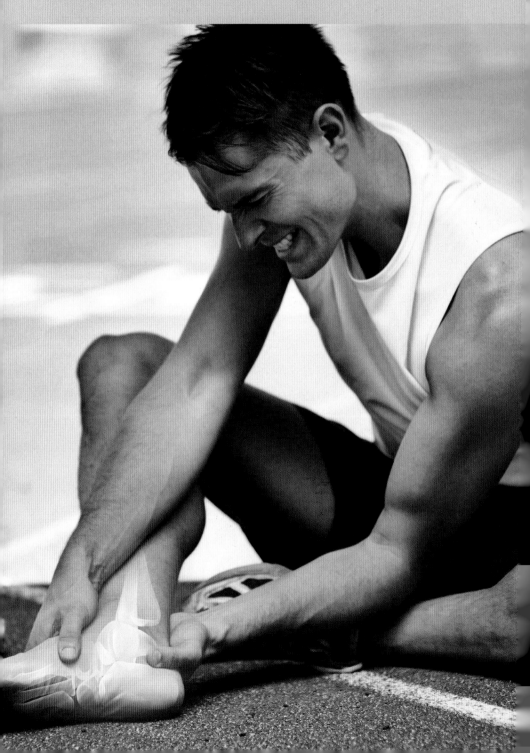

Injuries

'Stop training and rest your body!' A phrase most runners never want to hear . . .

Pilates for Runners isn't a book about injuries, although a lot of people only discover the power and joy of practising mat Pilates because they have been injured. Usually it's as a result of a referral by an injury specialist that brings about that first encounter with this form of exercise.

My osteopath/physio/chiropractor/sports therapist said I should do Pilates!' A phrase I often hear. . .

In this chapter you'll find information on common running injuries. I've listed the basic symptoms and usual causes, followed in some cases by expert advice and exercise suggestions. Obviously this isn't an exhaustive list, but these are the injuries I come across most often in my practice. This is only to provide guidance. Rather than hoping the symptoms will magically disappear and the injury go away of its own accord, I hope this chapter will encourage you to seek further, more tailored advice and help from a specialist. Once you know for certain what you're dealing with, you can begin to put things right.

I can't stress enough how regular Pilates can help you avoid injury. Having said that, the exercises can be equally beneficial if you are currently nursing an injury, helping you return to your running trainers rehabilitated and often in better shape than before the injury.

Acute injuries

Current thinking has now moved on from the familiar RICE acronym (Rest, Ice, Compress and Elevate) that has been applied to most acute injuries in the past. Research has shown that gentle movement with protection after an acute injury is more effective than complete rest. However, be sensible with this: if you are in severe pain when you start moving the injured area, then stop and seek specialist advice.

You will see I have used the acronym POLICE to replace RICE: POLICE stands for Protecting the area of injury, Optimal Loading (applying very gentle movement), Ice (10 minutes every hour), Compression and Elevation. The acute phase of an injury can be anything from 48–72 hours, or sometimes even longer. The time your injury takes to heal will depend on how serious it is and the location – the most pressing question every runner asks is 'When will my injury mend and when can I run again?' Or maybe it's the other way round!

Plantar Fasciitis

Symptoms

- Pain on the underneath of the heel sometimes likened to walking on glass, which is worse when you step on it first thing in the morning. As the fascia warms up the pain begins to subside.
- Discomfort can stop when you run but returns soon afterwards.
- If left untreated your gait will change to compensate for the discomfort and this can cause imbalances in the body.

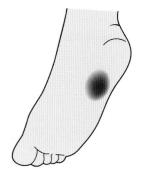

Plantar Fasciitis can feel like walking on glass

Cause

- Continual stress to the underside of the foot causing inflammation to the fascia and surrounding tissues.
- Tight Achilles tendons and/or calf muscles which puts more stress on the foot.
- Overpronation can put extra strain on the fascia.
- Worn out or non-supportive trainers can sometimes contribute.

Treatment

- Massage the underneath of the foot – roll your foot on a tennis ball, spiky massage ball, or over a small plastic water bottle filled and frozen.
- Ice the sole of your foot for 10 minutes after a run to help reduce inflammation.
- Night splints sometimes help, as do heel gels inserted in your shoes.
- Check that your footwear is correct – get your gait analyzed at a good running shop.
- Orthotics can sometimes help.
- Rest.

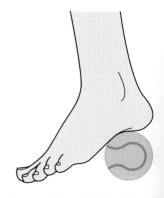

Massage with a tennis ball can help

Prevention

- Improve flexibility of the calf muscles and Achilles tendons – stretch well after and even during a run (page 166).
- Foot mobility and strengthening exercises (page 58).
- Pick up pens or small balls/marbles/towels with your toes to strengthen the feet!

ITB Syndrome

Symptoms

- Discomfort on the outside of the knee joint.
- Knee pain when running, particularly when running downhill.
- Pain in the knee area when straightening or bending the leg.
- Pain generally disappears when you stop running.

Illiotibial band

Friction against the femur

Cause

- Overuse. Inflammation is caused as the ITB tendon rubs repetitively over the outside of the femur (thigh bone) beside the knee, along with the constant knee-bending that running requires.
- It can also be caused by running off-road on uneven ground, or if your running technique and posture is placing stress on this part of your body.

Treatment

- Foam roller along the ITB band.
- Soft tissue massage of ITB, quads, hamstrings and glutes.
- Stretch all leg muscles.
- Ice the area.
- ITB stretch (page 167).

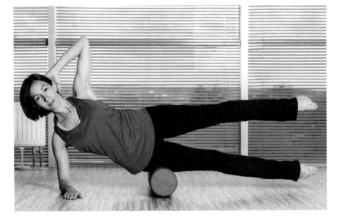

Prevention

- Work on your posture and pelvic stability.
- Regular stretching (see ITB stretch, page 167).
- Clam/Lateral hip opener exercise (page 98).
- Side Kick exercises (pages 88–101).
- Double Leg Stretch (page 122) to help strengthen and lengthen the ITB band.
- Wearing the correct footwear.

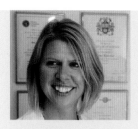

PROFESSIONAL ADVICE

Osteopath Jane Kaushal says that some of the common running injuries she sees include ITB, plantar fasciitis and Achilles tendonitis.

These are all linked with dysfunction of the posterior chain (glutes, hamstrings, calves). As with any injury, the part that hurts is only hurting because of a problem elsewhere. These posterior chain muscle groups need to be strong yet flexible for injury prevention and for rehabilitation to be as quick as possible. All this can be achieved by doing Pilates regularly. For example, the Clam exercise will significantly strengthen the glutes which will help to prevent/reduce inflammation within the iliotibial band.

Piriformis syndrome

Symptoms
- Pain deep in the butt!
- The pain can sometimes travel down the back of the leg and into the foot.
- Pain is worse climbing stairs or sitting down.

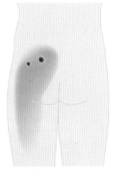
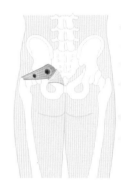

Piriformis syndrome

Cause
- Incorrect posture and running technique.
- Weak glutes.
- Tight adductor (inner thigh) muscles; the abductors (outer thigh) then have to work harder when you run, which means there is more strain on the piriformis as a result.
- The repetition of the running movement can sometimes shorten the piriformis group of muscles, which can cause the sciatic nerve to become irritated.

Treatment
- Deep tissue sports massage.
- Foam rolling.
- Piriformis stretching (page 165).
- Orthotics can sometimes help if pirirformis is due to overpronation.
- Rest.

Prevention
- Improve posture.
- Strengthen glutes (see Shoulder Bridge, page 125).
- Increase flexibility and strength of adductors (page 163).
- Piriformis stretch (page 165).

Achilles tendonitis

Symptoms

- Burning or tenderness in the Achilles.
- Pain and stiffness first thing in the morning with limited ankle mobility.
- Sometimes swelling and heat and a 'creaking' sensation.

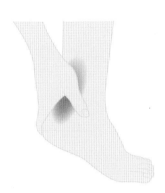

Achilles tendonitis

Cause

- Postural imbalances.
- Tight or weak calf muscles.
- Sudden increase in training, especially hill training or running on uneven terrain.
- Turning your foot over when running.
- Wrong footwear – lack of cushioning in the heel area.
- Overuse.
- Overpronation.

Treatment

- In acute phase apply POLICE.
- Gentle stretching of the calf (page 166)
- Gentle heel raises (page 57)
- Self-massage of the area and calf muscles to reduce tension.

Prevention

- Increase flexibility of the calf muscles and hamstrings.
- Muscle strengthening of the calf muscles and Achilles tendon (page 166).

> I have two on-going injuries, one is a groin (adductor) injury and the other is plantar fasciitis. There are specific Pilates exercises that form part of my injury management and rehab programme. For example, Pilates exercises to strengthen the glutes, hamstrings and adductors are helping me overcome the groin injury. Given the emphasis in Pilates for all-round strengthening of the body, it is hard to imagine that it wouldn't form part of an injury rehab programme.
>
> Tania Baldwin-Pask, trail runner

> Achilles tendonitis is often brought about by the runner neglecting to stretch. The shortening of the muscle increases the stress on the tissue and this is what results in injury. Stretching is usually very successful as a treatment and it is a good discipline to make stretching a habit after a run, but all too often it's rushed through as an afterthought. I encourage runners to participate in other activities to give variation in the movements that the body performs. Pilates is an excellent addition as it focuses on both stretching and strengthening.
>
> Simon Poole, podiatrist

Runner's knee (patellofemoral pain syndrome)

Symptoms
- General discomfort around the kneecap.
- Worse when running downhill or walking up and downstairs.
- Pain on bending the knee or squatting.

Cause
- Postural misalignment. – weakness in the hip abductors causing knock knees.
- Tight quadriceps, hamstrings, ITB and glutes.
- Overuse.

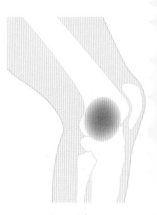

Runner's knee

Treatment
- Rest your knee! POLICE.
- Gentle stretching of the quads, hamstrings, calf muscles, ITB and glutes.
- Soft tissue massage or foam roller on the quads, hamstrings and calf muscles.
- Orthotics can sometimes help in the long term.

Prevention
- Single leg balance exercises (page 155).
- Quad strengthening exercises.
- Clam exercise/Lateral hip opener (page 98).
- Pelvic stability, quadriceps and glute strengthening exercises.
- Core strengthening exercises.

Shin splints

Symptoms

- Pain or throbbing in the front of the lower half of the leg, usually along the inner side of the shinbone (tibia).
- Worse at the start of a run, may ease off after a while.
- Discomfort returns when you stop running.

Cause

- Increasing mileage too quickly.
- General overuse.
- Muscle imbalance between the lower leg muscles and foot (tired or tight calf muscles).
- Running on hard surfaces.
- Incorrect footwear/worn out shoes.
- Overpronation.

Treatment

- In acute phase apply POLICE.
- Gentle stretching (page 163–171).
- Correct footwear with possibly more cushioning.

Prevention

- Warm up before running.
- Run on soft surfaces.
- Strengthen your lower limbs.

Shin bone pain

With all medical problems there are a number of ways a tissue may come under stress, and one of those may be due to the foot being in a position that places stress on that tissue. It could be that the foot is in an 'overpronated' position and as a result it is under stress. I have used inverted commas here as it is a misleading term because one person's overpronation may be much less than someone else's but gives them far more tissue stress. There is no norm or ideal position and it is about your body functioning within its tolerable limits. I do believe that attending a Pilates class is a very good way to keep your body functioning in its optimum postural position and as a result keeping you within your tolerable limits. If after this an injury occurs, orthoses may be the next step to get you back running again.

Simon Poole, podiatrist

Hamstring strain

Symptoms
- Discomfort or even swelling at the back of the thigh.
- Tightness in the back of the thigh when stretching the hamstrings or running.

Cause
- Increasing intensity of run too soon.
- Not warming up properly.
- Weak or tight hamstrings.
- Muscle imbalance between the hamstrings and quads, or weak glutes that have made the hamstrings work too hard leading to overuse.

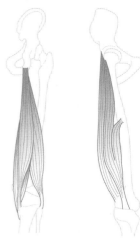

The hamstrings

Treatment
- In acute phase apply POLICE.
- Soft tissue sports massage when appropriate.

Prevention
- Warm up before running.
- Stretching and strengthening exercises.
- Shoulder Bridge (page 125).
- Side Kick exercises (page 88–101).
- Roll Down (page 53).

> Pilates exercises have helped to strengthen the areas affected by injury and have helped to keep other areas toned while I was waiting to run again.
>
> Marina Knibbe, self-confessed running addict

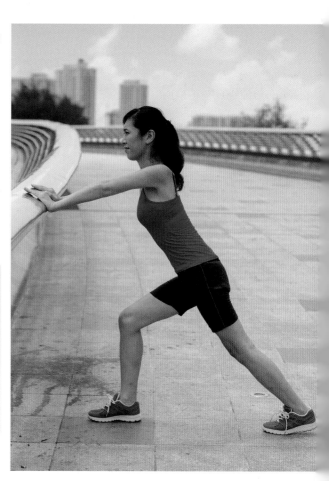

Calf injury

Symptoms

- Tightness or pain in the calf muscle.
- Finding it hard to continue running without pain.
- Swelling in the calf muscle.

Cause

- Not warming up properly before a run.
- Often a forceful contraction of the muscle.

Treatment

- In acute phase apply POLICE.
- Soft tissue sports massage when appropriate.

Prevention

- Strengthen the calf muscles (page 57).
- Lengthen and stretch the muscles.
- Warm up properly before a run.
- Single leg balance exercises (page 55).

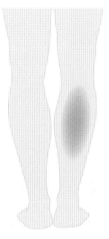

Calf muscle injury

The concepts and practice of Pilates parallels so much of what we aim for when applying soft tissue massage. By manipulating muscular and other tissues we hope to alleviate tension, 'snags' and other impediments to joint ranges, enhancing a person's ability to function and perform normal movement patterns, while helping with relaxation. Pilates promotes core strength, relaxation, mobility and balance, making it the ideal mode of recommended exercise following any massage treatment.

Tim Paine, author of *The Complete Guide to Sports Massage* and Director of Sports Therapy UK (www.sportstherapyuk.com)

Ankle sprain

Symptoms

- Pain and stiffness around the ankle joint.
- Swelling on the side of the foot.
- Discomfort on weight bearing and ankle instability.
- Bruising that moves down the foot.

Cause

- Turning or twisting the ankle.
- Running on uneven terrain.
- Tight Achilles tendon.

Treatment

- In acute phase apply POLICE.
- Try gentle ankle movements but make sure you don't increase the pain.

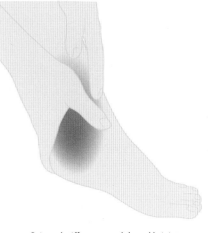

Pain and stiffness around the ankle joint

Prevention

- Strengthen the ankle joint (page 57).
- Single leg balance exercises (page 55).
- Core strengthening exercises.

It goes without saying that these injuries can quickly increase in severity if left untreated or ignored. Don't keep running – seek help. We runners are so bad at acknowledging injury and accepting that we need to stop. The pain is there for a reason, pay attention to it. In the long term the sooner you find the correct treatment, the sooner you'll be back running and not champing at the bit, worried your life as you know it has come to an end!

The tension caused by injury is in itself debilitating, both mentally and physically. Pilates can help you relax and hopefully relieve the anxiety and stress associated with being laid up. From a physical point of view, all the exercises support rehab as well as encouraging the muscles around the injured area to relax and let go, making it easier for the healing process to begin.

In addition, although I've mentioned a few specific exercises and stretches that can help in the prevention of some of the injuries, all Pilates exercises will of course help muscular imbalances through improving postural alignment and strengthening muscles.

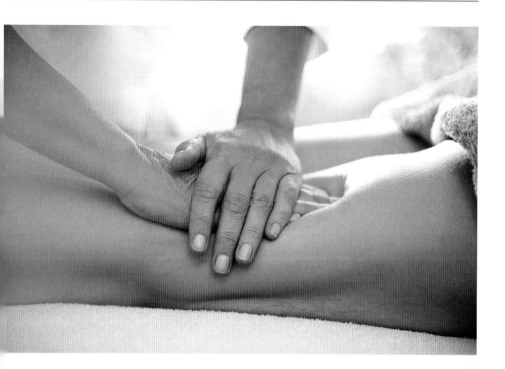

CASE STUDY

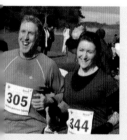

John Ford is a personal trainer from Norfolk who enjoys running anything from 5k parkruns to marathon distance. He has run four marathons and 30 half marathons.

I first started using Pilates to assist running injury rehabilitation and was immediately taken by how quickly it helped me to overcome injuries but also how it subtly developed additional strength. It has helped my endurance and those additional strength gains have helped me maintain running pace across a number of distances, despite the fact that at 62 I should be on the downward slope for race times. The regular use of Pilates exercises has helped me maintain form and I find in my age group at many races I am achieving better results than I did years ago.

A couple of years ago I was sidelined for a considerable time with a hamstring problem in my right leg, which developed into a further injury of my pes anserine below the knee. The physiotherapist I used was a Pilates instructor and apart from standard soft tissue treatment she added in a number of Pilates exercises to assist the rehabilitation. I now use these exercises as a matter of course in my running training routine.

All of my personal training sessions include a core strengthening phase. I believe it gives my clients an edge in their fitness that is not achieved by just conventional cardio and strength and conditioning programmes. That edge is in ensuring all of their muscles work well and work in sequence, it keeps them well and hence I think gives a confidence not achieved without the exercises.

Chapter 12

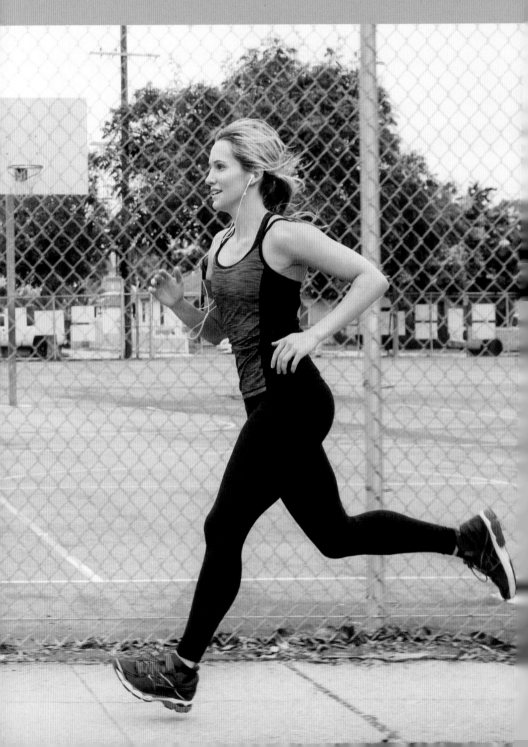

Pilates for the running mind

Anyone who runs, whether competitively, for health, fitness or for fun, knows that a huge part of the challenge can occasionally be just getting out of the front door. If the weather is wet and miserable and your 'to do' list feels endless, the challenge is no longer simply a physical one but also mental. Even though the legs are willing, the sudden lack of motivation can dramatically change your plans and play havoc with your training schedule. Not only that, but once you actually manage to leave the house and start your run, your mind can sometimes sabotage the enjoyment.

Take concentration for example, one of the Pilates principles you have been applying when practising the exercises (page 21). When you're running you should be able to focus fully on what you're doing, not allowing any negative thoughts to take over and distract. This can make the difference between gaining a personal best in a race or feeling completely demotivated and wanting to chuck your trainers into the next muddy ditch.

Even if you're enjoying what started out as a gentle stress-busting, endorphin-filled Sunday morning run, your mind can suddenly switch to work or family angst and ruin the experience. Keep your conscious mind on the job of running, let your unconscious mind sort out all the other stuff. The ability to focus on the right things at the right time is a skill, and by mastering this skill you'll discover that you can have a calmer and more fulfilling run. The knock-on effect is that your body will be happier too. As you learn to concentrate fully on the movements while practising Pilates, together with the balancing and breathing, you will find that your running concentration will improve. The more positive head space that Pilates encourages will also extend into your everyday life.

Some people find that a running 'mantra' or affirmation can help with focus, to keep them in the moment while they run. A mantra is a single word or a memorable phrase to concentrate on and repeat over and over. This repetition focuses the mind and prevents distractions and negative thoughts. These mantras are sometimes called positive self-talk and can be a very powerful tool. Choose your word or phrase and make it meaningful and reassuring to you; make sure it's not too long or complicated, so that when the going gets tough it just comes easily into your head and flows. Sports psychologists believe mantras allow the mind to lift itself out of

> A body free from nervous tension and fatigue is the ideal shelter provided by nature for housing a well balanced mind, fully capable of successfully meeting all the complex problems of modern living.
>
> Joseph Pilates

negativity and harness positive energy rather than dwell on failure or disappointment. Have a go – it works!

Another way to focus the running mind is to concentrate on your breathing, just as you do when practising the Pilates exercises in this book. Listen to your breathing when you're running, feel it, even count your breaths as a way of centring yourself and distracting your mind from any negative thoughts.

Relaxation, another of the Pilates principles, is worth consideration here. Research has demonstrated that if you are tense or overly stressed when running, you are more likely to suffer an injury. You might think that you are relaxed, but if your mind is distracted by worrying about something then you are likely to be tensing your body. Try to sense any areas of tension when you run – hone in on areas of your body and notice, if, for instance, your fists are clenched or your shoulders are up around your ears. This is where a check on your postural alignment comes into its own. Make sure that you're lengthening through your spine so that you feel lighter on your feet, your chest is wide and open and your shoulders down and stabilized. All this will have a positive effect on your mind.

Pre-race nerves affect many runners. The journey to the start of a race can provoke all sorts of anxieties: will you make it on time, have you checked your kit, will you be last, did you remember your race number or registration email? Getting stuck in traffic or getting lost and arriving with five minutes to spare can send your race body and mind into total turmoil. Then there are the numerous visits to the loo 'just in case' beforehand, and the checking and rechecking of race gels, shoe laces, Garmin charge and so on. It's no wonder that some people are prone to injury if they start a race in this state!

Standing with the pack at the beginning of a race is a good time to practise some Pilates breathing. Take a deep breath in through your nose and then let it out through your mouth – perform this several times. You can even close your eyes to block out the other runners around you so that you can fully focus on yourself. Go through your body and sense any tensions. Lift your shoulders up to your ears and take them down into your back pockets (page 33). Perform a few Roll Downs (page 53) and neck exercises, shoulder rolls, ankle circles, even stand on one leg to concentrate the mind. Devise a short relaxing ritual that you can carry with you to every race and you'll find that the wait at the start line will become a welcome time to centre yourself and become race ready.

When that long run or race is over, post-run Pilates exercises and stretches will relax your adrenaline-charged body and bring both your mind and body gently 'down' from the runner's high, enabling a better night's sleep and quicker recovery.

Pilates is a nice, relaxing form of exercise especially after long runs or high-intensity training. It also helps to lower my stress levels. I find it particularly useful after a race like an ultra marathon for removing any lactic acid as well as easing my stiff/sore muscles!

Jane Holt, ultra marathon runner

Chapter 13

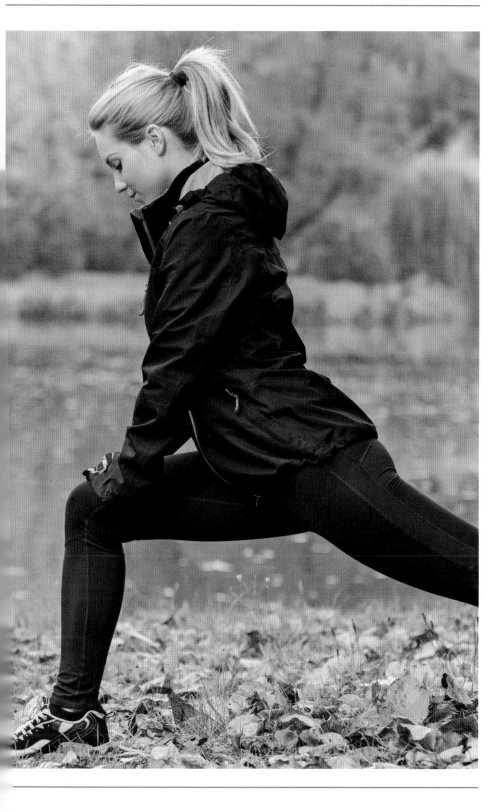

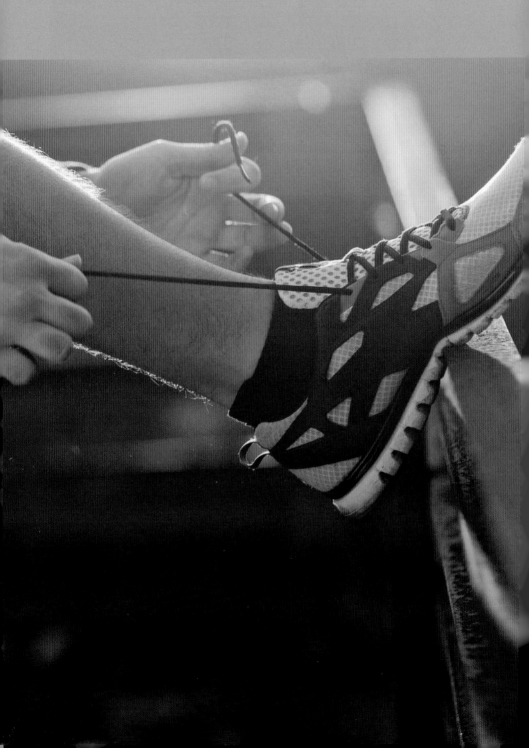

Finding a Pilates class: what to look for

All over the world, mat Pilates classes are part of the timetable of every health club and gym. Sessions are often very popular, but ideally there should be a maximum of about 12 people in each class. The reality these days is that there are a lot more people attending and so often the classes are oversubscribed.

If you are new to Pilates and have chosen to attend a class, ask the instructor to go through all the posture points with you beforehand to explain the 'Pilates language'. Although I've described everything I think you will need to know, each teacher will have their own way of explaining things. The instructor or health club should automatically check that you have no injuries or musculoskeletal problems and you will be asked to fill in a health questionnaire. If you do have problems then make sure the instructor is familiar with your injury and is happy to adapt the exercises to suit your individual needs. Or if your physiotherapist or sports therapist has recommended you try Pilates, it might be helpful for the instructor to have a letter or outline of your problems and what they advise. She/he will also check on what other exercise you do, your fitness level and why specifically you're choosing to come to a Pilates class.

During the class the instructor will stand in different parts of the studio and come round and correct, adjust and attend to you to make sure you are doing the exercises correctly and safely. She/he may demonstrate the exercises but won't be doing them all; his/her cues will be verbal and she/he will be constantly observing.

The first time you attend the class there's often a lot to take in. The music will be gentle background music and there should be space around your mat to move comfortably; you shouldn't feel jammed in like sardines in a tin. Ask questions – never feel you can't. If you don't understand what you're supposed to be doing, say so. A good instructor will welcome this and often there will be others in the class who might be a tad unsure too.

'The class I attend each week consists of mostly the same faces. Our instructor explains the moves really well in non-technical terms so easy to follow and usually has three levels of difficulty per exercise, which allows personal variation … like in the Shoulder Bridge, I like to hold the lift. I find it a great mix of being both very relaxing (I'm sure I fall asleep sometimes, I've certainly zoned out!) and great exercise … I find gyms boring but using your own bodyweight as resistance is neat.

Mark Burrell, marathon and ultra marathon runner

Pilates is a wonderful form of exercise and suitable for almost everyone: young, old, athletic, unfit, exercise phobic. For some, the hardest part is taking the plunge and going along to a class or talking with an instructor for reassurance. Happily, Pilates is at last now attracting more men as they discover the power of this form of exercise. For some men, and I know this from my clients, it's really quite daunting to walk into a class. But Joseph Pilates was a man, he created this extraordinary form of exercise for everyone. So really you have no excuse; equipped with the knowledge and experience gained from this book, all you have to do is sign up for a class. Combine a class and the exercises in this book and you'll be well on your way to staying injury-free and becoming a stronger, faster runner.

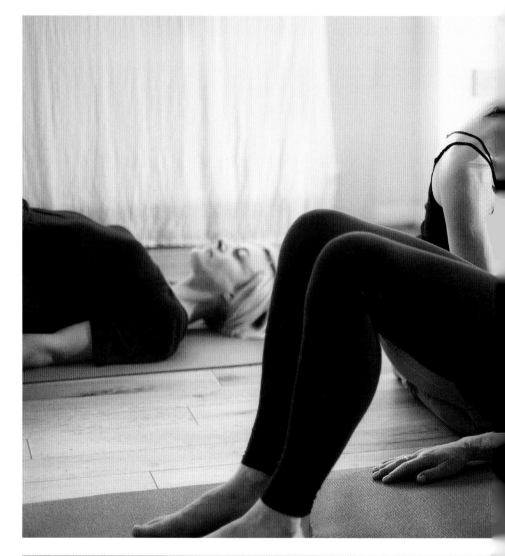

I have been teaching Pilates for just over 15 years and have had many sports people, including runners, attend classes. As Pilates helps strengthen the back and deep abdominal muscles, my clients report that they are able to run up hills more efficiently. They say the exercises have increased their stamina as they are able to use their diaphragms properly and experience less tension in the neck and shoulders. Clients become more body aware and so are able to focus on proper movement with better awareness, leading to less strain on the body and injuries.

Sarah Pyle, mat Pilates instructor and sports therapist

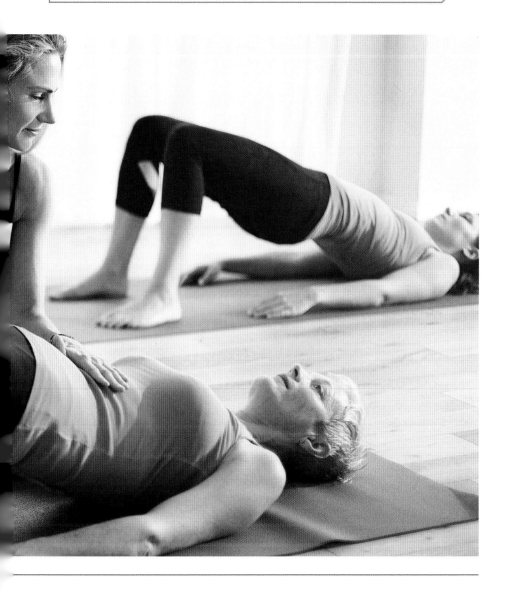

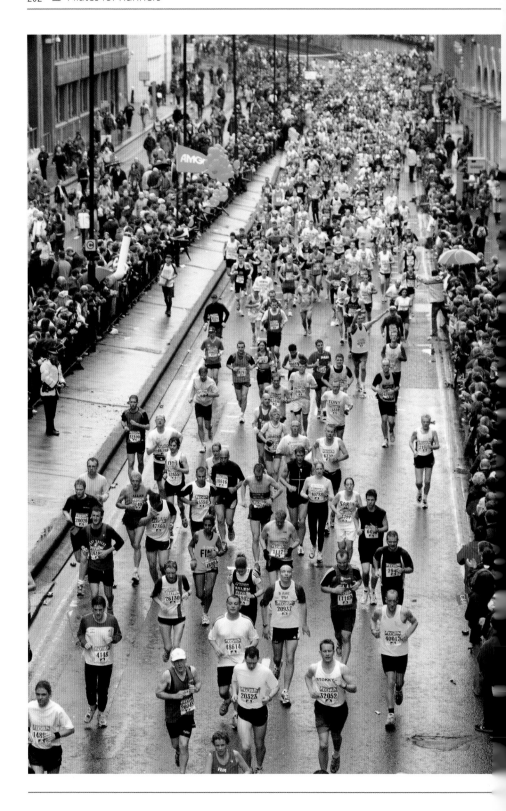

Acknowledgements

An especially big thank you must go to all my clients, friends and fellow runners who contributed to this book, and those who continue to inspire me and make teaching Pilates and running so life-enhancing.

Thank you to the 'experts': Jane Kaushal, Simon Poole and Dr Helen Kennedy for their invaluable input and wisdom.

And of course Charlotte, Sarah and the team at Bloomsbury for their support and guidance.

About the author

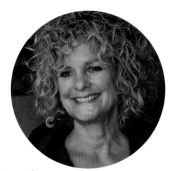

Harri's running career almost ended before it started over 30 years ago, when she could be found scantily clad, flouncing around Hyde Park and falling over a lot. Fast forward to 2007 when she entered her first London Marathon and took up mat Pilates. She was hooked. For Harri, Pilates and running are a way of life now; she couldn't live without either.

To date she has run eight marathons, including one ultra, many half marathons, 10ks and 5ks, and thanks to Pilates doesn't fall over any more or flounce. She leads local running groups with the unfortunate acronym of HRT (Harri's Running Team) and is passionate about helping people to start running and fulfil their goals whatever their age, size or fitness level. Harri's Running Team has featured in both *Women's Running* and *Running Fitness* magazines.

Harri is a REPS level 3 qualified mat Pilates instructor, personal trainer and UKA leader in running fitness. She works out of her own private exercise studio in Marlow, Buckinghamshire, where she teaches regular weekly mat Pilates classes and sees private clients. She has written for *Running Fitness* magazine as a roving reporter, and lives with her husband, on and two border terriers.

You can follow her on Twitter @harriangell or contact her through her website: www.runwithharri.co.uk.

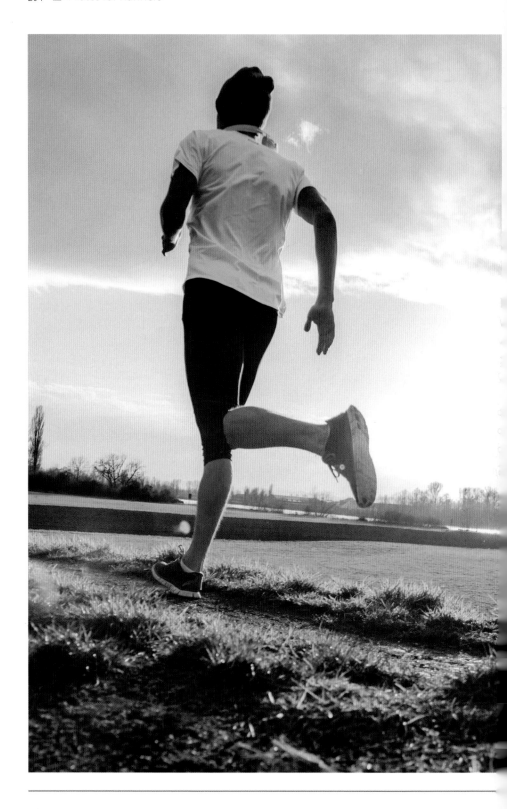

References

Page 11:
Kimitake, Sato and M. Mokha (2009) 'Does core strength training influence running kinetics, lower extremity stability, and 5000 –M performance in runners?' *Journal of Strength and Conditioning Research*, 23 (1): 133–140.

Page 12:
Published by ChiroAccess Editorial staff (2010) <http://www.chiroaccess.com/Articles/Preventing-Sports-Injuries-through-Proprioceptive-Neuromuscular-Training.aspx?id=0000142> Accessed 29/09/2016.

Page 13:
Alison McConnell, quoted by Brian Dalek (2013) <http://www.menshealth.com/fitness/secret-to-running-faster?_ga=1.173098080.2109377137.1475161404&fullpage=true> Accessed 29/9/2016.

Page 13:
Phrompaet, S., Paungmali, A., Pirunsan, S., Sitilertpisan, P. (2011) 'Effects of Pilates Training on Lumbo-Pelvic Stability and Flexibility', *Asian Journal of Sports Medicine* 2 (1) 16–22.

Index